THE

Mother-to-Mother

POSTPARTUM DEPRESSION

SUPPORT BOOK

THE

Mother-to-Mother

POSTPARTUM DEPRESSION

SUPPORT BOOK

*Real Stories from Women Who
Lived Through It and Recovered*

SANDRA POULIN

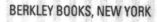
BERKLEY BOOKS, NEW YORK

THE BERKLEY PUBLISHING GROUP
Published by the Penguin Group
Penguin Group (USA) Inc.
375 Hudson Street, New York, New York 10014, USA
Penguin Group (Canada), 90 Eglinton Avenue East, Suite 700, Toronto, Ontario M4P 2Y3, Canada
(a division of Pearson Penguin Canada Inc.)
Penguin Books Ltd., 80 Strand, London WC2R 0RL, England
Penguin Group Ireland, 25 St. Stephen's Green, Dublin 2, Ireland (a division of Penguin Books Ltd.)
Penguin Group (Australia), 250 Camberwell Road, Camberwell, Victoria 3124, Australia
(a division of Pearson Australia Group Pty. Ltd.)
Penguin Books India Pvt. Ltd., 11 Community Centre, Panchsheel Park, New Delhi—110 017, India
Penguin Group (NZ), Cnr. Airborne and Rosedale Roads, Albany, Auckland 1310, New Zealand
(a division of Pearson New Zealand Ltd.)
Penguin Books (South Africa) (Pty.) Ltd., 24 Sturdee Avenue, Rosebank, Johannesburg 2196, South Africa

Penguin Books Ltd., Registered Offices: 80 Strand, London WC2R 0RL, England

This book is an original publication of The Berkley Publishing Group.

"Heart to Heart" reprinted with permission from Dr. Charles R. Solomon, *Handbook to Happiness*, (Tyndale),
www.gracefellowshipintl.com.

All Scripture references are taken from the King James Version of the Bible, unless otherwise noted.

Berkley trade paperback edition / March 2006

Library of Congress Cataloging-in-Publication Data

Poulin, Sandra.
    The mother-to-mother postpartum depression support book : real stories from women who lived
through it and recovered / Sandra Poulin.—Berkley trade pbk. ed.
      p. cm.
    ISBN 0-425-20808-7
    1. Postpartum depression—Popular works. 2. Postpartum depression—Anecdotes. 3. Postpartum
depression—Patients—Biography. I. Title.

    RG852.P65 2006
    618.7'6—dc22   2005057062

10 9 8 7 6 5 4 3 2 1

PUBLISHER'S NOTE: The events described in this book are the real experiences of real people. However,
the author has altered their identities and, in some instances, created composite characters. Any resemblance
between a character in this book and a real person therefore is entirely accidental. Every effort has been made
to ensure that the information contained in this book is complete and accurate. However, neither the publisher
nor the author is engaged in rendering professional advice or services to the individual reader. The ideas, pro-
cedures, and suggestions contained in this book are not intended as a substitute for consulting with your physician. All matters regarding your health require medical supervision. Neither the author nor the publisher shall
be liable or responsible for any loss or damage allegedly arising from any information or suggestion in this
book. While the author has made every effort to provide accurate telephone numbers and Internet addresses
at the time of publication, neither the publisher nor the author assumes any responsibility for errors, or for
changes that occur after publication. Further, the publisher does not have any control over and does not as-
sume any responsibility for author or third-party websites or their content.

The Mother-to-Mother Postpartum Depression Support Book *is dedicated to all the mothers who participated in this book, as well as all mothers who have recovered from postpartum depression and are openly sharing their experiences to help future mothers recover. . . .*

And to my precious daughter, Rachel Lilly, who is the greatest joy of my life.

Acknowledgments

As I was walking on the treadmill this morning, my daughter, Rachel, proudly displayed her latest artwork that she had just finished coloring with crayons. Her picture, called "Postpartum Depression," featured three women sitting on a bench in a park, with their babies on their laps. Sprinkled around the picture were happy and sad faces, and colorful rainbows. What a masterpiece!

Now, I realize that most nine-year-olds are not drawing pictures with postpartum depression as their theme. But Rachel's experience growing up has included a mommy who juggles both motherhood and career (as so many mothers do), plus, always "Mom's book project."

Little by little, year after year, *Mother-to-Mother* has been in the making, and now the two most important people in my life, husband, Tim, and daughter, Rachel, are sharing in the joy of the book's completion. I hope this process will encourage and inspire Rachel to always reach for her dreams!

While I suffered from postpartum depression, I had so much wonderful support to help me recover. Kenneth Price, Ph.D., Neal Sklaver, M.D., and his nurse, Nancy Avila, are excellent, compassionate medical professionals.

Gloria "Sita" and the late Myron "Papa" Krasno are amazing parents who cared for both Rachel and I 24/7 at my lowest hours. As it happens, "Sita" has spent most of her professional life as an advocate for the mentally ill, and "Papa" was a "natural nurturer," so I was in the best of hands. Jeannine "Mopsy" Poulin is the kindest mother-in-law a woman could ask for. She is always there for us and is the "rock" of her family. Melissa Bennett, then our live-in nanny, was more helpful to my recovery than she'll ever know.

Terri Cohee and Lisa McIntosh, your help on the Participant Biography forms was key. Susan and Alan Brown, David and Lisa Roebuck-Krasno, Cindy and Joel Vardy, Caren Krasno and Doug Cohee . . . all family who I counted on.

Special thanks to Bradley Richardson, my mentor through the publishing process, and Robin Weaver Conley and Linda Harwood for helping with the typing. My website was managed by brilliant friend Vonn Zauber, who, together with Patti Zauber, is what my father would have described as a "giver."

Debbie Estrin, James and Annette Flick, Gordy and Wendy Hoover, JP and Gail Martinez, Damon and Carol Oran, Dory and Ira Petsrillo, Ron and Sherry Zander . . . you are the best and most supportive friends. You have stood by me through all the ups and downs in this book-writing process, and have been instrumental "Aunts and Uncles" in Rachel's growing years.

Jane Honikman, thank you for all your support while creating this book . . . and for devoting your life to building Postpartum Support International into a strong, worldwide organization that women combating this illness can count on.

Finally, thank you to my agent, Marcy Posner, and my editor at Berkley Books, Christine Zika. You believed in my book. You understood how healing *Mother-to-Mother* could be for so many women in the future. I will be forever grateful to you.

Contents

Foreword

Sometimes language confuses us. In the vernacular we say "postpartum depression" or "PPD." More accurately, PPD is called Postpartum Mood and Anxiety Disorder or Major Depression with a Postpartum Onset. But PPD also includes emotional reactions during pregnancy and after adoption. It refers to a continuum of mild to severe symptoms, from the baby blues to psychosis. The complexity of these definitions can keep women from finding the help they need. This book alleviates this confusion because mothers describe their own experiences with PPD.

Women like to talk. We feel a need to share our experiences and compare them with others' experiences. This is especially true as we encounter pregnancy, birth, and child rearing. I believe this sharing is a natural and critical aspect of being a healthy individual. It allows us to learn from the past and prepare for the future. It is known as *Mother's Wisdom*.

There is a universal message that I share with the mothers and their families who contact me about postpartum depression. I want them to know that 1) they are not alone, 2) they are not to blame, and 3) they will be well. They are not alone because at least 10 percent of pregnant and postpartum women will be affected. They are not to blame because most probably this is an inherited illness. They will be well because depression is very treatable. This is true. Sandy Poulin has produced a landmark book that addresses each part of this universal message. She has given mothers an opportunity to share their stories as loving proof of these truths.

The voices in Ms. Poulin's *The Mother-to-Mother Postpartum Depression Support Book* represent every imaginable emotional experience related to childbearing. While each woman's experience is unique, it contains common threads of a similar fabric. These include pain and joy, fear and hope, despair and exhilaration, illness and wellness. There cannot be a "right way" to be pregnant, give birth, and recover. Our bodies—and that includes our brains—perform in mysterious ways. We must talk about these phenomena with other women who have "been there." This is especially true for those of us who have experiences I describe as "less than wonderful." The emotional side of motherhood is the least described and discussed. Society is uncomfortable with the collision of the motherhood myths and mental illness. Denial, ignorance, and stigma keep PPD a silent and neglected disorder.

I am asked, "Did you have PPD?"

"Yes," I reply.

They respond with, "Tell me about your experience. How long did it last? How many children do you have? What did you do to get well?" These questions are examples of a woman's right-to-know. She is searching for information, on a quest for answers. She is saying, "Tell me the truth."

- Why am I feeling these strange sensations?
- What is happening to my mind?
- How will I ever be "myself" again?
- When will I sleep again?
- Am I a bad person?

The insights gained and expressed by the mothers in this book are powerful. Their words provide validation, reassurance, hope, and emotional support. They represent the wisdom gained from the terrifying journey from health to illness and back to health again. Everyone who cares about the future of our families should read these stories.

Professionals can provide psychotherapy and medications to treat PPD, but it takes the mother-to-mother experience to truly learn about being well again. I commend the courage of these mothers who have shared their stories and I thank Sandy Poulin for giving them a voice through the pages of this book. It is an important contribution to our Postpartum Parent Support Movement.

—Jane Honikman, M.S.,
Founder, Postpartum Support International

Introduction

I was on top of the world! The baby I longed for, ached for, and prayed for, had finally arrived. My husband and I were blessed with the daughter of our dreams. After enduring three years of fertility treatments, our in vitro attempt was successful. My daughter was born perfectly healthy, and I was so grateful, so ecstatic. Little did I know that just four months later, I would be in the depths of postpartum depression.

Welcome to *The Mother-to-Mother Postpartum Depression Support Book*. If you are experiencing postpartum depression and are looking for women who have recovered, you have found us! I hope that knowing recovery is possible is in itself a great relief to you. Although hundreds of thousands of women in the United States, and millions worldwide, experience postpartum depression each year, actually finding a mother who will admit she had it and who is willing to talk about it is very difficult.

After all, most of us survivors know firsthand the pain when a family member or friend in whom we've confided reacts with shock and dismay. I actually had someone tell me that my postpartum depression must be God's way of telling me that I wasn't supposed to be a mother. Scathing reactions such as this illustrate that there is still stigma and shame surrounding this illness. But how can anyone who hasn't battled it truly understand the devastation of being utterly exhausted to the core, yet completely unable to sleep? The torturous sleep deprivation, the tremendous anxiety, uncontrollable crying spells, and the loss of control. Worst of all, the fear that we might never recover. People who haven't experienced this just cannot fathom how a mother who has just been blessed with the greatest gift of all—a new human being—could possibly become depressed. Well, none of us expected to feel this way either . . . and none of us wanted it.

It is estimated that only one in three mothers seeks help for postpartum depression and only about twenty percent of cases are actually diagnosed. The vast majority of mothers with PPD—as will be shared through stories in this book—believe that they shouldn't feel bad after giving birth. Our society and the media portray new motherhood as a time of great happiness and joy, so these new mothers feel shame and fear being stigmatized—labeled—as unfit mothers. They would rather hide their symptoms than admit them to family, friends, or even their physician.

After Andrea Yates drowned her five small children, postpartum depression and psychosis gained worldwide attention. During this time of intense interest in this illness, many women bravely talked with the media about their experiences. But the Yates tragedy is the type of extremely rare event that cloaks postpartum illnesses with such stigma. Cases like these make the news, of course, but in reality the vast majority of mothers who suffer from postpartum depression never harm themselves or their babies. In fact, they will fully recover and enjoy motherhood.

This book is not about the "whys" of postpartum depression. I am not a medical professional, and there are many great books available written from a clinical perspective. No "wading through" medical jargon or research studies here. This book is different. It is from mothers, to mothers. Pure support. Real stories from cover-to-cover. It is the book I searched for when I had postpartum depression, but could never find. What I did find were some great medical postpartum depression books, sprinkled with real-life examples. Reading these brief gems gave me the most relief. These mothers recovered, and so could I. It was these few and far between stories that gave me the most hope. "Most books about postpartum depression are very informative about the illness," as one mother explains. "But what I need, as someone who now suffers from PPD, is not risk factors, theories about its cause, or prevention tips. These things are useless once you are in the throes of depression. I need to read about other women's experiences and what I can do for myself." Exactly. This is why *Mother-to-Mother* was created.

Once I recovered, I began to devote all the time I could muster outside of my busy family life and career to create this book. I utilized new mother magazines and the Internet to find mothers who wanted to participate in this project. All of these mothers felt the same passion I did. We've all survived and have gone on to enjoy our lives again and relish our roles as mothers. We all wished we had a book just like this one to help us recover.

After an acquaintance of mine learned about my book she asked, "Why would you want to go back *there*?" Mothers with this view may want to "sweep PPD under the rug." But every time I received a story from another mother who was eager to participate, I knew we were on to something. We believe this "grass roots" book will help to validate our feelings and experiences, and provide reassurance for mothers to recover.

If you are reading this book to increase your knowledge about postpartum depression, you may be startled by the mothers who had hurtful thoughts toward their babies. I'm grateful I didn't have this symptom, but please do not condemn these mothers as bad mothers. Although these entries may provide the most troubling aspect of this book for readers (and they certainly caused the most pain for mothers experiencing these thoughts), they were just thoughts. Even if you have never experienced postpartum depression, there is a good chance someone you know, love, and respect has had it. The hurtful thoughts and other symptoms are from this biological medical condition that none of us ever expected or wanted. In fact, most of us had never even heard of postpartum depression, because it was so rarely talked about. For a long time most of us didn't even know what was wrong with us until we were finally diagnosed.

If you are a medical professional, I hope you will learn from our shared experiences the importance of diagnosing postpartum depression as quickly as possible, before an overwhelmed mother falls into the lowest depths of despair. Although some of us had a bout with clinical depression at some time in our lives previously, many of us never experienced depression until our postpartum period. And it is crucial for those in the medical community who "don't believe in PPD" to become educated about this very real illness. Thankfully, celebrities, including Brooke Shields and Marie Osmond, are bravely sharing their stories and should be congratulated for helping to educate the public about postpartum depression.

If you are now experiencing postpartum depression, this book, which has taken many years and many moms to create, is just for you. Feel free to read it from the beginning to the end, or simply open up the book in a time of need, see where the pages fall open, and read from the mother who "is there" to help you. Each mom's story has just a couple of pages at most to keep it as easy as possible and user-friendly for exhausted, sleep-deprived mothers to read. Some of the entries shared in this book represent the first time these mothers have had the courage to express themselves—sharing experiences they said they haven't even told their best friends.

Although several mothers were so passionate about this health issue being brought out in the open that they *did* want their names used with their stories, I nevertheless changed all names to protect their identities. Each mother's story contains intimate, raw details of her postpartum depression experience. You may not relate to every symptom, but you'll know that we all recovered after—in many cases—deep despair. Then you'll read about our accomplishments and/or thoughts now that we are well again.

You'll find a wide variety of inspirational stories and quotes from other mothers. Many are grouped together into chapters named for the mothers' most prominent symptoms. You'll find my story first, followed by stories of mothers in similar life events in the postpartum period. But many symptoms and life experiences overlap . . . so some stories could have easily found a home in several chapters.

Most of the mothers who participated in *The Mother-to-Mother Postpartum Depression Support Book* sought professional treatment from a psychiatrist or psychologist, and were prescribed antidepressant and sleep medications. I cannot stress enough how crucial therapy and medication were to their recovery and I urge you to consider seeking help from a qualified professional.

I hope you will identify with some of these mothers, many of whom have offered some personal tips that have helped them recover. Rest assured that you are not alone. I wish I had the space available to include every single story that was submitted to me. I am forever grateful to all the mothers who entrusted me with their stories. Become strengthened from so many wonderful women around the world whose combined wisdom has made this project so fulfilling. You will find only brief comments from me . . . I prefer to let all of our mothers speak for themselves.

So, pull up a cozy chair, and snuggle in it with your baby (or wait until baby is sleeping if you like), and grab that box of tissues. This time I hope your tears will flow from relief, from hope, and from the mother-to-mother love that leads to healing.

Sandy's Experience

RADIO ADVERTISING SALES EXECUTIVE (AUTHOR)
TEXAS, USA

In February of 1996, my daughter, Rachel, was born. After enduring several years of extensive fertility treatments, including a successful in vitro fertilization and frozen embryo transfer, I delivered a beautiful, healthy baby girl. The baby I ached for, prayed for, and desperately wanted to love and nurture was finally in my arms. I was ecstatic. I fell instantly and deeply in love with her. Little did I know that just four months later, I would come to experience the depths of postpartum depression.

Over the next year, I would experience the lowest, most frightening period of my life. I was completely unaware that there was even an illness called postpartum depression. But I knew that something wasn't right. I was having difficulty sleeping. I heard how sleep deprivation could result from infant feedings. But even when my daughter slept through the night, I could not. I was extremely "keyed-up," feeling a great need to check on her often to be sure she was breathing and okay.

During maternity leave, I felt very isolated at home. My husband traveled for his job and was only home on the weekends. I was accustomed to talking to dozens of coworkers and clients every week, and now that I was home with my baby, all day and all night,

I didn't realize how much I needed the people contact and the daily structure of work. I was so alone. It was a tremendous adjustment to be home during maternity leave, away from my fast-paced career. I was questioning who I was . . . a business executive or a mother. I was always driven to be the best I could be—a classic perfectionist—and now as a mother I worried if I could be either.

After yearning to become a mother for so long, I expected this period to be the happiest of my life. But night after night I could not sleep. I loved breast-feeding Rachel, the miracle of it . . . I loved the nurturing feeling of providing her milk, I enjoyed the sensuality. However, after becoming exhausted from sleep deprivation I felt as if my last bit of precious energy was being drained out of me through breast-feeding.

As I became more sleep deprived, I became overwhelmed with worry that I could not function any longer. The days seemed so long. I lost track of time. I was so tired; it seemed a monumental task just to take my baby to the grocery store. I started to cry often. I began to lose my appetite. I lost my ability to think clearly. As the sleepless nights added up, the tears and anxiety started to increase at a faster pace. I realized that something was terribly wrong. I made an appointment with my therapist, the same excellent doctor who had seen me through the only bout of clinical depression I had ever experienced—ten years earlier, after I contracted mono. He began leading me through relaxation exercises as a technique to help me sleep. But I wasn't sleeping yet.

Adding to my worries, I knew I needed to return to my high-pressure work environment as a radio advertising sales executive. We needed the money and my job share partner, also a new mother, was becoming anxious for my return.

Four months after Rachel was born we prepared to leave for our annual family reunion. It took every ounce of energy I had to pack for the trip. My husband drove us to the airport and got us on the plane. My parents knew I was not doing well. One look at me and my mother knew that I was an empty shell. She found a wheelchair for me at the airport and transported Rachel and me to the car on four wheels. My parents intended to fortify and heal me before the arrival of the rest of the family two weeks later.

Those two weeks were a trip through hell. Despite using the pre-scribed sleeping pills from my family doctor, I still couldn't sleep. (By now I was weaning Rachel off nightly breast-feedings so I could safely take sleep medication.) The medication would put me to sleep for just one or two hours. That was it. Once I was awake, I cried all night long from a complete inability to shut off my racing mind. Night after night crying spells consumed me. My mother mothered me as well as Rachel as I was just incapable of dealing with her.

I started to have suicidal thoughts. I was petrified of them—I had never experienced this in my life. My mind was out of order. I felt as if my mind was a pinball machine "on tilt." In fact, some-times I felt possessed. To cope with the relentless and surreal image of putting a gun to my head, I would "fight it" by pulling the trig-ger in my mind and forcing myself to create the vision of a bouquet of flowers popping out. It was the only way I could control the ending—because these visions took control of my mind with their random occurrences. The flowers in the "ending" gave me the only hope I had. I talked to my parents about hospitalizing me, but they said I wasn't ill enough. Little did they or my therapist know I was having vivid suicidal thoughts hour after hour.

While still under my parents' protective wings my mind tried desperately to zero in on a solution as to how to care for my infant and help my shattered mind heal. I made urgent phone calls to my husband to locate a nanny, as I did not feel up to the task of caring for our child. I was worried I was losing my mind.

When the rest of the family arrived for the reunion, they were thrilled to meet the newest addition to the family. I was relieved to have so many family members "love her up" and watch over her while my mind was broken. I still did not realize that I was in the depths of an illness with a name. I was hanging onto the threads of my sanity while my days were filled with three-hour crying spells, feelings of panic, and knots in my stomach. I couldn't eat. And worst of all—I couldn't sleep.

In an ultimate act of desperation, I pulled aside my sister and my sister-in-law and asked if either one of them would raise my beloved daughter were I to end up in a mental institution. This was so beyond what they thought I would ever say that their reaction was shocked silence. How could Sandy—the type A, competent, successful business executive who was always in control and organized—be asking such a ridiculous question? They giggled as they talked about the possibilities of who should take Rachel. They didn't understand that this was the most important and difficult request I had ever made. How could they not see my pain? They tried to make a joke of this. It was a question I would never forget, as I fully believed that I would or should end up in some sort of hospital.

The trip home was filled with unspoken dread. How could I cope? Who would help me? How could I care for Rachel? After our return, my therapist was able to see the extent of my illness. He diagnosed me with postpartum onset depression. What a revelation! There was a name to attach to the hell I was going through. I was finally empowered to start to learn about this illness.

I was fortunate to have been in a job share situation and in a company that was very supportive of my needs. Luckily my job share partner was able to work full-time to cover for me until I was able to return. Along with my job share partner and medical documentation, the job got done and I was able to delay my return to work.

For the next several weeks, I cast about looking for help. Had anyone ever suffered through this illness? Was there any advice? How had they dealt with this? Had any medication helped them sleep?

An old friend called me one day as a result of hearing of my search. She had discovered that one of her friends had suffered from postpartum depression and was willing to talk to me—a complete stranger—about it. She strongly recommended an anti-anxiety medication for sleep. I suggested this medication to my therapist and eventually he did prescribe it to me. This was finally the medication that allowed my mind to sleep.

I have a distinct memory of a session with my therapist during which he said he was impressed that I had been so proactive in trying to find help for myself. That struck me . . . how could anyone in this terrible state of mental illness not seek out any and all help they could to climb out of this dreadful place?

Our "nanny search" was successful, and we used our emergency savings to hire a young woman. She ended up living with us for a full year and her companionship was instrumental in my recovery.

The first night on the anti-anxiety medication I fell into a deep sleep. While I slept, our nanny and my husband paced the house worrying and talking, worrying and talking. They worried that I had been overprescribed. All I did was sleep! I remember the incredible relief I felt when I woke up. I was thrilled from the rest. I was also fearful that this was some sort of fluke. Would I sleep the next night? The next night the medication worked again and I slept soundly. After two nights of medicated sleep, I had hope. For the first time in five months, I thought that I might recover and get back to normal again. I believe that anti-anxiety medication saved my life.

My husband and our nanny took turns with baby "night duty" while I took the medication every night to catch up on my sleep. Over the next year I slowly recovered with the tremendous support of my husband, family, medical professionals, nanny, and antidepressant and sleep medication.

Eventually, I was weaned off the medications and could finally sleep on my own. The crying spells lessened and I started to think clearly again. My positive, enthusiastic nature was resurfacing. I slowly regained energy, rebuilt my confidence, and climbed out of that utterly debilitating depression. I went back to work and it would take a full year to recover.

When I told my husband that I no longer needed our nanny to live with us, he said, "I finally have my wife back!"

Now That I've Recovered

Our nine-year-old daughter is the center of our life. I love being a mother, but what a rocky start! Now, when I see a new mother pushing a baby stroller in the mall or at the pediatrician's office, I can't help but wonder if she's suffering. Having PPD was one of the scariest periods of my life, and it sparked a deep passion inside me to create this book to help mothers recover.

> Take walks by yourself. I would take walks with my earphones on, listening to my favorite uplifting songs that I had my husband record on my "happy tape." These walks were without the baby, who I'd leave with my husband or nanny. Walking to this upbeat tape helped revitalize my health and spirit and made me feel much more confident about myself again. I've always loved music and I responded well to my "music therapy."

I had excellent health care through fertility treatments, pregnancy, labor, and postpartum. I had plenty of support from many friends, clients, and family. And I have a happy disposition. If PPD can happen to me, it can happen to any woman.

PPD must become more openly talked about. It must be diagnosed quickly to prevent or lessen the severity of this painful illness. Perhaps someday posters will be displayed in all OB/GYN and pediatricians' offices. The poster could say, "New mothers, are YOU having trouble sleeping?" And it should list symptoms of PPD and contact numbers for help. This poster would be seen by new mothers taking infants to "well baby" visits and could be used as a preemptive strike against PPD. Along with "well baby" visits should be "well mommy" checkups to be sure postpartum mothers are coping well.

Heart to Heart

When we come to the place of full retreat
And our heart cries out for God,
The only person whose heart ours can meet
Is one who has likewise trod.

Others may offer a word of cheer
To lift us from despair;
But above the rest, the one we hear
Is the whisper, "I've been there."

—Dr. Charles R. Solomon,
from *Handbook to Happiness*

CHAPTER 1

Mothers Overcoming
Sleep Deprivation

When I was pregnant, the advice I heard most often was "get your sleep now—before baby arrives" and "sleep when the baby sleeps." The advice would be followed by giggles of parents who knew that unless you've ever been through new parenthood you couldn't possibly understand how hard it is, those first weeks and months, from sleep deprivation. After all, many babies want to stay awake all night long or be fed.

Now I wonder . . . are those words, so commonly said to future mothers, a universal "warning system" of what may be coming along with that bundle of joy? Nobody wants to be negative to a pregnant woman and alarm her about the possibility of postpartum depression striking. So the "get your sleep now" advice could be as close as well-wishers dare say about what trouble might be looming in the forecast.

The mothers' stories in this chapter—and indeed in the entire book—reflect that the interrupted sleep pattern night after night took a terrible toll on their postpartum selves, both physically and mentally. Insomnia was absolutely the most common symptom from all the stories these mothers shared; therefore I'm starting out the book with stories that stress this symptom. Whether a mother couldn't get back to sleep after a midnight feeding, woke up way too early with that sense of dread of facing the new day without nearly enough sleep, or like me, couldn't get to sleep altogether, we all would find that the method or medication to help us sleep was a turning point toward recovery.

After baby arrives, most new mothers hear the following from well-wishers: "Is your baby sleeping through the night yet?" But the question I always ask a new mother—in a gentle voice—with her baby in the stroller at the grocery store or mall is: "Is Mommy sleeping through the night yet?"

~ AMELIA ~
34, TEACHER
CALIFORNIA, USA

I expected big demands and sleepless nights, but I never imagined I would feel the way I felt. At two and a half weeks postpartum, I literally stopped functioning. My severe sleep problems were the most disturbing symptom. I wanted nothing more than to sleep, but I was too riddled with anxiety to relax. Even after taking pills to sleep, I'd wake up at three A.M. and would immediately feel the anxiety as though I had not slept at all. I felt incapable of mothering a baby. I felt my life was over, that I was losing my mind, and would either end up dead or institutionalized.

Although my family was reassuring, I feared they'd eventually tire of taking care of me and listening to me repeat the same worries over and over. I couldn't talk about anything other than my crisis. All other issues seemed so trivial. All my thoughts and energies were devoted to figuring out how to survive. I moved into my parents' home and my mother became my son's primary caretaker. I cried so often and feared anyone could just look at me and tell I was mentally ill. I couldn't get enough reassurance that this condition wasn't permanent, and the reassurances I did receive didn't mean anything to me unless they came from a mother who'd "been there." And I couldn't find any of these moms. Many did talk of the baby blues, but I was always quick to point out that they were able to function one way or another. I had shut down entirely. I didn't want to die, but I thought that taking my life was something I might be forced to do as a last resort, to get relief from the pain.

At first I received help from a therapist, then a psychologist. They both assured me this would all just go away. They didn't seem to comprehend the seriousness of my frame of mind. Then a family friend recommended a psychiatrist. I was prescribed an antidepressant, which I took for a year. A persistent friend of mind discovered "Depression After Delivery" and had them mail me information. I cried tears of relief as I discovered other women who had survived PPD to the degree that I had it. I read that pamphlet over and over when I needed it.

The only thing that kept me sane was knowing that others had PPD and had made it through. I searched desperately for anyone with my symptoms to reassure myself that I, too, would one day have my life back and be happy to be alive. By far the most help came from former sufferers.

EMMA
AT-HOME MOM/BUSINESS OWNER
CALIFORNIA, USA

I didn't realize how bad the sleep deprivation would be or how constant my baby's crying, and how I couldn't do anything else besides care for the baby. I heard all of this, but didn't grasp what it would mean day to day. I had to beg my mom to help, and she gave me only a few days. She thought I should be able to handle it on my own. After all, she did. Then when PPD was diagnosed, she came back—reluctantly—for two weeks. I became ill at childbirth and at three weeks stopped breast-feeding to take an antidepressant prescribed to me. It took two more months to start feeling better and seven months to totally recover.

I had severe insomnia. I wouldn't sleep for four to five days at a time. I had to take twice the maximum recommended dose of sleeping pills and sometimes along with it an antipsychotic drug prescribed by my doctor to get even a few hours of sleep. I felt very weak, emotionally vulnerable, and fragile. My husband was doing all the night feedings. I was totally overwhelmed and scared that the intense anxiety would stay with me and I'd never enjoy being a mother. It was emotionally painful to spend time with my child—it is very hard to convey this feeling. I thought I was going crazy since I couldn't sleep, and sometimes I would hear things that weren't there. I wasn't hallucinating, just suffering from lack of sleep, but it was spooky.

I felt that my body and mind were breaking down, like a car running out of fuel. I wasn't sure how much longer I could survive (whether my mind or body would give out first). Really, I lived in a state of despair and fear for my mental condition. I remember buying an excessive number of diapers at one time, as I was concerned I'd get stuck without some and run out at the last minute. This unpredictable event left me scared, although it seems silly now; but I think my life was so out of control that I couldn't handle even a minor surprise such as this! I really felt like I was living a nightmare, and sleep offered no solace.

I felt bad about myself, but I tried to remind myself that this PPD was beyond my control and that a "good mom" was still inside of me. I couldn't shake that "sinking" feeling in the pit of my stomach, which I took to be extreme despair. It lasted continuously for two months.

I saw a social worker who wasn't that helpful. I knew more about PPD than she did. I saw another therapist who I didn't like—he treated PPD clinically, and was not very supportive. I found a psychiatrist who acknowledged the uniqueness of PPD—he was the most helpful. I had never believed in antidepressants before, but the medications he prescribed were the reasons I survived. Second to the drugs was the support of my husband, my mom, and a volunteer from a PPD support group I attended a couple of times. I concentrated on trying to lead a regular life, which was very hard.

Thoughts for a Better Day

Although there's a stigma about taking medication, I encourage moms to be open-minded. The drugs are temporary until the body/mind can work itself out. It is important to get help right away and not let PPD drag on. In the end, less damage is done if it's treated early. I also avoided being around new mothers who were "oohing" and "aahing" that everything was great. I found older moms with more perspective very comforting. Just focus on getting through each day, not too much into the future.

> You aren't alone. This is not your fault. You will be well again. This is treatable. Keep repeating this like a mantra; it will make you feel better.

MADELINE
33, MAGAZINE EDITOR
NEW YORK, USA

I knew mothering wasn't going to be easy, but I didn't know it would be this hard. Every move had to be thought out. Even just taking a shower required major planning and maneuvering. What hit me hardest, though, was the lack of sleep. People warned you about that, and I always said, "Yeah, yeah," but I did really miss my sleep.

My head swirled with all the questions I had—about bottles, about poop, about all the noises he made while he slept. I was too wound up to sleep. Everyone tells you about the wonderful feelings involved with being a mother, but no one tells you about the down side. It's like a big conspiracy. No one would ever have another baby if the truth came out.

I remember looking at other mothers with babies—searching for any sign that they were having as much trouble as I was, but all they would do was smile, kind of a Mona Lisa smile, and go on strolling with their babies. I felt very alone, like a terrible mother. A friend of my sister's had to be hospitalized after the birth of her first child because of depression, but it was sort of talked about in hushed tones, and we all thought that this woman was a little "neurotic" and just couldn't handle the pressures of motherhood. Little did I know that I would be speaking to her just a month after I had my baby, talking about feelings and experiences that we had in common.

My husband and I grew closer. He was wonderful and really took care of the both of us. He hoped I'd eventually snap out of it, but while he was away on a business trip I told him on the telephone that I wanted to give the baby away so we could just go back to the two of us. There was a long pause on the line and he said, "Okay, I'm coming home tomorrow."

He checked all the Internet PPD sites he could find so he had a real understanding by the time he got here. I was so depressed that I couldn't even pick up my son. It was a vicious cycle: The more I avoided my baby, the less I knew about him and the less confident I felt.

Another time I remember my mother asked me what I wanted for dinner and I actually became angry because it took too much out of me to make that decision. I thought it was terribly inconsiderate of her to ask me that now. Yet, before my baby was born, I was in a high-powered position, working on deadlines and making quick decisions. Now choosing dinner was too much.

I was consumed with my baby's little world and nothing else. Time was suspended. The world had stopped. Or more like I just wanted the world to stop so I could rest. My husband took me to the emergency room during an anxiety attack, and I was relieved to be admitted for a few days of rest. The psychiatrist there was the first person who helped me feel normal in weeks. He assured me my illness was common and treatable. He also referred me to a therapist and I had about ten sessions with her. Medications were prescribed and I started to feel better after about two weeks.

Thoughts for a Better Day

I've gone back to work part-time and I feel great about that. Since I've gotten through this, I think anything else should be a piece of cake. I'm not scared of things anymore. After that horrible experience, I'm actually thinking of having another baby, which is proof that you can get through something like this. If only a tiny part of you can believe it, that's a start.

> Plan to do one thing out of the house each day. Go to the store, go for a walk, or meet someone for lunch. This one thing will help shape your day.

‑‑‑‑ BEVERLY ‑‑‑‑
41, EDUCATOR K–5
CALIFORNIA, USA

When my daughter finally started sleeping six to eight hours at a stretch, I still couldn't sleep a wink. She was four months old, and the severe lack of sleep was turning me into a complete wreck. At one point, I realized I hadn't had any sleep for three entire weeks. None. Not even a five-minute nap. I couldn't eat, had panic attacks, and thought I was going to die. I was afraid of everything and had no idea what was going on with me. Unless you've been this stricken with anxiety and terror, there's no way anyone can really empathize. When I went to a new moms' group and saw all the moms cooing happily about how great everything was, I dropped out of this "support" group. I was so jealous. I even started looking through the phone book at adoption agencies and imagined giving her away, and what a relief that would be. It was during this time that my husband later confessed that he thought about taking our baby and leaving me.

I found a counselor who specialized in postpartum depression. She saved my life. I will be eternally grateful to her. I was such a mess—I couldn't drive. She started helping me on the telephone. She put me in touch with other mothers who recovered, and that gave me hope. She connected me with a psychiatrist who prescribed medication for me. I was very close to being hospitalized, but managed to respond quickly to the medication and support.

Now That I've Recovered

My wonderful daughter is five years old, and I'm very happy I didn't give her away! I'm fine and glad to say I sleep soundly every night and feel thankful for my blessed life. Postpartum depression is completely hormonal/physical and can happen to any woman regardless of her personality. The last thing a sufferer needs is to feel like she had something to do with it. *Remember—you are not to blame for this. Don't blame yourself and don't take blame from others.*

ᵕᘐᕀ Monica ᘐᕀᵕ
28, At-Home Mom
Pennsylvania, USA

My doctor told me to expect a "bout of sadness." He gave me some pamphlets, but, of course, I didn't think PPD would happen to me. My family and friends couldn't believe I had postpartum depression because I had such a good baby.

Although I was "weepy" for the first three months postpartum, I don't think the depression started until about three months after delivery. It lasted a year. I had trouble sleeping at night and never could nap during the day. I ate like crazy. Even though I had "baby fat" to lose, I couldn't stop. Food was my friend and was always there for me. I would cry at anything and was paranoid my husband was having an affair. I cried because I was crying and couldn't just get a hold of myself. But when I was in front of people, I was an actress, hiding everything. I began to think that I was not a good mother or wife. That made me think about ending my life, but I would worry about who would love my baby as much as I did and take care of her.

Now That I've Recovered

I joined our local chapter of the National Association of Mothers Centers. When I began to seek out other mothers who gave up working for the "glamorous life" of a stay-at-home mom, I began to realize that I made a great choice and that the isolation that I felt didn't have to be there. I started a home-based business. And my marriage is better than ever!

> God could not be everywhere and therefore He created mothers.
>
> —*Jewish proverb*

➝◉ PORTIA ◉➝

35, AT-HOME MOM
ALBERTA, CANADA

From day one I had problems sleeping. No matter how tired I was I couldn't nap when the baby did. At about ten weeks postpartum, I honestly did not sleep for two weeks. I got to the point where I was scared to bother going to bed at night because I knew I would not sleep and would be absolutely frantic by morning. The baby's sleeping was not an issue at all. She was doing thirteen to fourteen hours a night!

Everyone around me was scared to say or do the wrong thing, whatever that may be, and they walked on eggshells. I now know the power of hormones and how, when they are grossly imbalanced, they can do amazing things to your brain—affecting how it functions.

A lot of times I felt like I was asleep and my head was on automatic pilot—but the pilot was some sick, demented, cruel thing running the show (my brain). At my lowest—when I hadn't slept for two weeks—I begged my husband to take me to the hospital so they could put me to sleep with drugs. I thought I'd be put in a psychiatric hospital and that my baby wouldn't know me. My mind just would not shut down—not relax for one second.

My brain was in overdrive and it was so scary, not having control over it no matter how hard I tried. I was not the same person anymore. I just wanted so badly to be myself again. But no matter how bad I got, I knew I would not hurt my baby.

I went to a psychologist and antidepressants were prescribed. After about two weeks, the drugs helped and in eight weeks I started feeling much better. I was finally becoming rational enough that I could start to write thoughts in a journal. The good days began to outnumber the bad. I relied on my husband, my mother, and mother-in-law, and definitely the medication. It took six more months until I recovered.

Now That I've Recovered

I had never been so scared in my life. But with PPD, I thought I might never have my "self" back. Now I am stronger for having gone through this and surviving it. I don't take anything for granted now: family, friends, clean air, nature, love, food, our home, even our mental health.

Thoughts for a Better Day

"I know now that motherhood is a journey. The gradual transformation of a woman into the person God intended her to be. It is not an easy job, but one with unmatchable rewards. Remember, becoming a mommy is probably the biggest change you'll ever go through. Give yourself time. Give yourself patience. Even women who didn't have postpartum depression did struggle in the beginning."

—Sasha,
British Columbia, Canada

CHAPTER 2

Mothers Overcoming
Fear and Anxiety

Any change in life can produce stress and anxiety. What bigger change occurs in life than the addition of a new baby? Unfortunately, too many mothers who only expected this time to be filled with joy will instead become excessively worried, are unable to relax, and even suffer panic attacks.

The mothers in Chapter Two express a variety of fears, from someone stealing their baby to Sudden Infant Death Syndrome. Mothers with postpartum depression suffer a variety of fear and anxiety symptoms while adjusting to the realization of the enormous permanent responsibility in their new life.

Their joy is released as they also share the happiness they feel after overcoming their fears and anxiety on their journey back to wellness.

‑‑‑ CLAUDIA ‑‑‑
32, AT-HOME MOM
ONTARIO, CANADA

The depression hit me six weeks postpartum, following weeks of crying jags. I was incredibly emotional and had mood swings that almost paralyzed my husband with fear. He couldn't understand what was happening. I didn't make sense to him. He would tell me to lay down, get some sleep, but it never worked.

If it hadn't been for some articles I read, I wouldn't have identified the problem. My husband and I just clung to each other and hoped it would get better. We stayed close and suffered together. I would hold my screaming baby and sob, crying as I walked with her. I cried a lot . . . felt dull . . . with a dull headache . . . dull life. With the exhaustion, fear, and sadness I felt like a zombie that was only around to deal with the crying and needs of a baby. I walked through it in a numb state, feeling guilty while attending to my daughter and not enjoying it.

I withdrew from my close family and friends, thinking they wouldn't understand or believe me. The anxiety attacks were severe. I was given medication to put under my tongue to calm me rapidly. These attacks were the hardest symptoms to deal with. In my mind I was a complete write-off, not even resembling my old self at all. Eventually I had a complete breakdown before seeing a psychiatrist and getting medications, as well as counseling.

I think my psychiatrist saved my life. Also, I found relief at an Internet PPD support site. Reading other moms' problems and responses was an integral part of my recovery. The warmth was incredible, and I cried a lot with gratitude because I'd found others out there with the same problems. I no longer felt alone. Ultimately, I relied on myself to get stronger, better, and well. I went deep inside myself, and pulled all my internal strengths together to fight for wellness. Even in the bleakest moments, I relied on my own belief that I would get well.

Now That I've Recovered

I am a good mother who looks forward to the future. I have a new attitude toward mental illness, and can be more empathetic to others now. I look at both sides, not just my own perception. Also, I now understand how fragile the human mind is, which I believe makes me stronger. Stay away from people who don't think PPD exists. They are out there and this is not your fault. Use support from others to help you through.

> For I the Lord thy God will hold thy right hand, saying unto thee "Fear not, I will help thee."
> —Isaiah 41:13

EMILY
28, PURCHASING OFFICER
QUEENSLAND, AUSTRALIA

I had insomnia in all shapes and forms. Couldn't nap with the baby, couldn't sleep at night, and when I did, I had nightmares. As sleep deprivation wore on, I lost control of my body and emotions. No one, I believed, could possibly understand all of this.

I had constant fear of everything. I couldn't relax. I was in a deep hole and couldn't even find the first rung on the ladder to climb out. I've always been a bit moody, but this PPD was just crazy. I felt numb. Food made me nauseous. It took all my strength to eat a yogurt or a piece of fruit. I could have stayed in one spot and never moved again. I was so physically exhausted and emotionally drained I felt my body was made of lead. When I started to have hurtful thoughts toward my baby I immediately sought help.

Through a local mental health service, I found a psychiatrist and was prescribed an antidepressant. Months later, when I was cleaning house with a stomach virus to prepare for visitors for my daughter's christening, it hit me that our home was never perfectly clean before the baby, so it didn't need to be now. I realized that I'm allowed to feel bad and not feel guilty about it. As I began to recover, I set tiny goals—even one goal a day (wash nappies)— and slowly I increased the goals. Finally I started weekly goals, then monthly goals. It helped me feel organized and in control again. I also found that I had better days when I was out of bed by 9 A.M.

Thoughts for a Better Day

More than ever, I appreciate what I have in life. As the saying goes, the more pain you feel, the more joy you can know. This is not a road that I chose to travel, but it is one that has taught me so much. I would never change having a child for anything.

If you have PPD, and feel alone, don't worry about the phone bills. Reverse the charges if you have to. But call someone: your mother, sister, or friend. Talk about it. I had to do a lot of talking to get through this.

Ask your family, friends, and husband what you are doing well. You may be surprised to find that what you perceive you are doing poorly, everyone else thinks you are handling just fine. This will help you realize you are a good enough mother, which really means you are a perfect mother just the way you are.

᙭᙭ MEREDITH ᙭᙭
38, AT-HOME MOM
ENGLAND, U.K.

When my son was four months old, it was suddenly apparent that all was not well with me. I was frightened to go to sleep because I thought I would die. I was afraid to be alone—not only in the house but in a room by myself as well. I was even frightened in the bathroom.

My mother came to live with us when my husband went back to work. I was too scared to stay in the house, but terrified to go out, too. I had panic attacks all the time, for no apparent reason. Every time something hurt I thought it was fatal. I had pains in my legs and thought they were blood clots that would circulate to my heart and kill me. When I had indigestion, I thought it was a heart attack.

I managed to do the absolute minimum—feeding, dressing, and bathing my baby—but I never enjoyed him at that stage. Even now, many years later, I still don't know what I was terrified of. I had trouble eating and sleeping, but staying awake was hell. One night after admitting my deathly fears to my husband, we went to see the doctor. He diagnosed me with PPD and sent me to a psychiatrist. The therapy sessions did not seem to help me much, although for some people it's the best thing they can have. The antidepressants, however, helped me from day one. The first night I took them I slept better and regained my appetite.

Now That I've Recovered

What actually helped me more than anything was talking to other people and discovering I wasn't alone—that I would not end up in a straight jacket in an asylum. The more I was able to talk, the better I began to feel. Slowly, very slowly, I began to regain control of my life. For every two steps forward there was one step back and sometimes I despaired that I would never become "normal" again.

A sound machine, turned on to the nature sounds, can make your home soothing and very relaxing.

I started to face my fears and stay home alone. I started inventing errands for myself, such as to get a pint of milk. As long as I had a target, I could arrange to get out. Slowly the forays led me back into the big, wide world again. I didn't panic as much and there were more good days than bad. My son is now three and I have a five-week-old baby. Admit it if you have PPD and find support. You will get better!

⤳ ARIEL ↢

33, FILM AND TV MUSIC MANAGER
CALIFORNIA, USA

My PPD started in my second week of motherhood and lasted three and a half months until the antidepressants really started working. I was so anxious I lost my appetite and all taste, rapidly losing over thirty pounds. I had no interest in anything. Decisions about what to eat and wear were even too hard, so I did the same thing everyday: I ate a banana and yogurt and wore jeans and a black shirt. I was sure my husband was going to leave me because I was so down, not at all the "go-getter" I normally am.

I shopped around for a psychiatrist and therapist who specialized in PPD, and I had a very tough time with the antidepressants first prescribed. But after several medications we found the one that worked. I felt better after six weeks. They were miracle drugs! It was hard to stop breast-feeding and I felt guilty about it, but I feel that a happy non-breast-feeding mother is better than a miserable one.

Now That I've Recovered

I think my marriage is stronger than ever because now I know I can completely depend on my

> Make friends on an Internet PPD support group. Emailing them every day can make you feel better. Don't suffer alone—get linked together on an Internet PPD support group.

husband. While in the middle of the depression I didn't think I would ever get out of "the pit." Once I recovered, I knew if it ever happened again, I would recover again.

⁓☙ FELICE ❧⁓
27, AT-HOME MOM
NORTH CAROLINA, USA

I didn't have unrealistic expectations of new motherhood. I had worked in child care and knew how demanding babies were. Plus, mothers in the past had shared their stories of new motherhood with me. And yet, about two weeks postpartum I started to feel overwhelmed. My mind was going 100 miles per hour all the time about all that I had to do to be the perfect mother. I constantly worried I was doing things wrong, and that I had made a mistake by having a baby.

I slept okay at night, but I could not catch up on sleep during the day, when my daughter napped. I was always nervous about her waking up. I totally lost my appetite and had to force myself to eat. Also, I was very irritable and emotional, crying a lot. If I wasn't crying, then I was just numb. I knew sleep deprivation was involved. I was so tired I was never ready to face the day. I didn't feel capable of taking care of her, although I knew I could never hurt her. Still, I felt guilty about her being gassy and in pain. I felt all my anxiety was being passed to her through breast-feeding. Because I was such a nervous wreck and couldn't eat well, I thought this hurt her through the milk.

My husband went to the library and checked out a couple of books. One listed all the symptoms I was experiencing and I realized I had PPD. I went to see my OB/GYN and I was prescribed an antidepressant by a psychiatrist. After taking it for two weeks, it kicked in. Once the drug started working, I was a totally different person. It leveled off all the anxiety and worry. I also started taking walks, setting daily goals, and giving myself positive self-talk. And I prayed to God for inspiration.

Now That I've Recovered

I have a wonderful, healthy, and smart little girl. I know she's so smart because I stay home with her and teach her. I enjoy watching my child and seeing her accomplishments. I have come so far that I want another child. I'm scared of getting PPD again, but at least this time we will know what it is and how to treat it.

When I have bad days, praying to God gives me strength. Don't feel as if you're alone. PPD is a common problem that can hit anyone. Don't be afraid to get help, and don't be ashamed either. You will get through this.

Thoughts for a Better Day

View your experience as a passage in life . . . a chapter in a book that will end only to lead to a new beginning. What is happening to you psychologically and physically are only symptoms of an illness that will pass once it's run its course. You can handle this; otherwise you wouldn't have it. Be tough, be strong, and do whatever it takes to get well. Help yourself first, and then you will be able to help others.

Be very open with your doctor. You are helping both yourself and your baby. And remember, there will be a day that you will help make the difference in someone else's life through sharing your experience.

—Jordan, Advertising Executive
Pennsylvania, USA

CHAPTER 3

Mothers Overcoming Thoughts of Suicide and/or Infanticide

Mothers who suffer from postpartum depression know that probably the most distressing symptoms of the disease are the scary, obsessive thoughts and images that flash in a mother's mind. Terrifying thoughts of harming herself and/or her baby. I can't stress enough that these are unwanted, unwelcome thoughts. These mothers emphatically express that they love their babies . . . so why on Earth would these images surface? They are only thoughts, not actions, but they cause tremendous guilt, shame, and confusion to mothers afflicted with them. These women had no idea where these thoughts came from or how to stop them.

As you can imagine, mothers rarely shared their visions with others for fear of being misjudged as unfit. The mothers in Chapter Three bravely shed light on these tormenting symptoms, which they said made them feel "out of control" and led them to fear they were "going crazy."

Once they sought out professional treatment, they realized that postpartum depression is a medical illness and they were not to blame. Know as you read these stories that like all the other mothers in this book, these women offer their very own personal experiences to validate any of the same feelings you may be having—to assure you that with treatment you can recover.

⟶ OPHELIA ⟵
37, ARTIST/FLORAL DESIGNER
MASSACHUSETTS, USA

About two weeks after my baby was born, I began to feel terrified. I had a constant fear that something bad would happen to him. I couldn't look at our set of knives. I moved them so I wouldn't see them. I would notice that the baby would fit in the oven. I was plagued by visions of horrible things happening to my child: of him falling out a window . . . you name it. I was repulsed by these thoughts. My heart would thunder in my chest from terror.

I still did my best to care for my son and I didn't tell a soul about the thoughts because I was afraid of being called an unfit mother. I breast-fed often because he was a hungry baby; and I was constantly exhausted. He was not a good sleeper. My husband was very supportive throughout all of this. He took good care of us and was a proud daddy. But this all affected our sex life. Prior to childbirth I really enjoyed sex. It would be almost fourteen months before my husband and I had sex again—and I never felt the same about it.

Although I had spells of depression and had used antidepressants in the past, this time I suffered in silence. I was militantly committed to medication-free breast-feeding. Ten months postpartum I finally saw a social worker. Two months of seeing her made me realize I needed to see a psychiatrist. I stopped breast-feeding and began taking the prescribed antidepressants. Once I started sleeping and getting my energy back, I started to exercise and make new friends at church.

Now That I've Recovered

Our marriage is strong. I love being a mommy and a part-time flo-
ral designer. And I'm pregnant again. This time I have a plan. I will
not breast-feed, so I can get adequate rest (my husband will bottle-
feed at night). My doctor is ready to prescribe antidepressants
quickly to try to fend off the depression. And I will not isolate myself, but stay in touch with my mommy friends. Most of all, if
things start getting really bad again, I'll contact my psychiatrist and
nip PPD in the bud.

REBA

27, AT-HOME MOM

CALIFORNIA, USA

I had no idea how "touched out" I would be by the end of the day.
The constant holding, breast-feeding, cuddling, and touching the
baby made me fantasize about being naked in a dark room with
nothing—not even clothes touching me. Not a good thing to be
thinking about when your husband comes home from work.

My postpartum depression started two months after my baby
was born and lasted seven months. When I started investigating
postpartum depression in child-care books, there was a lot of mis-
leading information. Many devoted a measly paragraph to it and
flippantly discussed baby blues and postpartum depression together. But there is no comparison of blues to depression.

I could barely sleep. I waited for my baby to wake up, checked
to see if he was breathing, and breast-fed when he woke up. And I
cried all the time. An outing to the grocery store took normal preparation plus mental preparation for me. I'd tell myself, "No crying
for the next half hour so your eyes aren't so puffy. You can do it." I
wanted to tell my husband about my horrible thoughts of abandon-

ing or hurting my baby, but I was afraid he would leave me. I was such a basket case. My frequent thoughts of leaving my baby in the trash or tossing him off the balcony caused me to hate taking the garbage out, and I kept the balcony door double-locked. I knew I would never do these things, but I was fighting to stay sane. The awful thoughts and guilt made me feel like I was going crazy.

I joined a parenting class for infants, and I think it saved my life. I met other women who were feeling some of the same things. When I slowed down my nursing at eight months, I started feeling better and more optimistic. Once I stopped nursing, my old pep came back, and I started feeling my normal self again. As I started making friends in the mothers' group, my new friends commented on how fun I'd become.

> Cast thy burden upon the Lord, and he shall sustain thee. He shall never suffer the righteous to be moved.
>
> —Psalm 52:22

─────── SERENA ───────

31, EXECUTIVE ASSISTANT

HOLLAND, THE NETHERLANDS

I had irrational thoughts and was convinced my daughter didn't like me. It felt like my daughter was an "intruder" in my life and I feared I would never really love her. I had terribly scary thoughts of throwing her down the stairs. I flirted with suicide while driving. I'd think, "If I drive into the river, this will all be over."

I was lucky . . . my daughter was born in a hospital where an authority on postpartum depression in The Netherlands works. At my six-week postpartum checkup, my OB/GYN saw what was going on and managed to get this psychiatrist to see me at once, so I didn't have to "shop around." Once I was diagnosed with an actual condition—postpartum depression—I had great relief. Before that I was just convinced that this was what motherhood was like and that there was something wrong with me for not feeling blissfully happy. Now I could fight this. . . . It could be treated.

It took four weeks for the antidepressants to begin to kick in. I slowly began to make a daily schedule and add routine and structure in my life. I've climbed out of that black pit. I'm back to work, and organizing a conference for our company. Most important, I adore my daughter. But what a difficult start.

Now That I've Recovered

If you have postpartum depression, you know like I do that your life—as it was before you became a mother—is over. I think we are allowed to mourn every now and then. No one can go through such a life-changing event without suffering from shock. Allow yourself to feel that way and give yourself time to get comfortable with your new life.

⤳ WHITNEY ↢
31, EDUCATIONAL ASSISTANT
ONTARIO, CANADA

At first I was unable to sleep because I was breast-feeding every four hours, but then I was unable to sleep because I was suffering anxiety attacks in the middle of the night. I remember feeling absolute terror when nine P.M. would roll around. I was staying at my parents' house and everyone worked. I would take the baby upstairs as if I were going to my death sentence. At least during the day I had people to talk to or even just be with. Once nine P.M. came I was basically locked up in my bedroom with the door closed and no one to talk to.

I spent the night alone, trying to breast-feed the baby (I had problems with it), get him back to sleep, and worrying about his weight gain. It was hell—there's no other way to put it. I thought I was a horrible mother. Here was this beautiful baby boy that I had wanted for so long and I didn't care. He deserved a "good mother" and was stuck with me—frightened, anxiety-ridden, unable to care for him. I remember sitting in the park thinking all the logical things that I might tell myself: "Snap out of this . . . you're lucky you have him, you wanted this baby for so long, he's a beautiful child and you're being ungrateful for this gift." If someone had come and taken him from my arms, or if I dropped him and walked away, I wouldn't care. I felt so horrified at this and sat and cried and cried with this little baby in my arms. I believed I was the worst mother in the world and didn't deserve to have this baby.

When I realized something was very wrong with me I called our family physician. Eventually, I was prescribed an antidepressant by a physician. I stayed on it for fifteen months. It helped me greatly. Looking back, if I had to do it again, I would have quit breast-feeding and taken antidepressants right away. The emotional quality of your relationship with your child far outweighs the benefits of breast-feeding.

Now That I've Recovered

The saying "hit rock bottom" sure applied to me. I also managed to deal with my husband's leaving me, after he was home for nine days, when the baby was eight weeks old. He said the baby "got on his nerves," and he didn't want the responsibility. I've learned to get help when I need it. When I stopped pretending everything was okay and admitted the PPD to others and myself, only then could I begin the road to

> Keep a journal. When angry or frustrated, stop what you're doing and write until the anger and frustration go away. This is not for anyone else's eyes.

recovery. It was not until then that friends admitted that they had endured it, too. That's the thing that I couldn't understand. Why had no one ever mentioned it? It was almost like a deep, dark secret that only those in the know could be told about. The information I had read did not prepare me for the depths of PPD. I now have much more empathy for others and I'm also a dedicated mother to my son. I've begun a new relationship. I enjoy life again.

~~~ YVONNE ~~~
28, AT-HOME MOM
TEXAS, USA

For two years prior to my son's birth, I was a social worker for at-risk new mothers who lacked support and resources: no education, no significant others, nothing. I was educated about PPD. I knew the importance of having a support network, but somehow felt one was only necessary for those in great need. I often felt it was selfish of me—a college graduate with a very supportive husband and bank account—to ask for support when many women seemed to manage with so little. And I believe that in my family it was acceptable to give help, yet not acceptable to receive it. I withdrew from all family and friends. . . . I didn't want to have to explain to anyone that I was depressed, and I didn't want anyone to judge me or disagree with the way I felt.

The moments I found myself falling asleep behind the wheel especially concerned me. My most vivid, painful memories are the violent thoughts of throwing my baby across the room . . . immediately followed by uncontrollable sobbing, increased sadness, and frustration. I suffered from panic attacks when visiting others, because I risked "exposing" my depression. I had suicidal thoughts. In the deepest depression, I felt certain my husband and son were better off without me.

I received no professional help or medication. It may sound trite, but I relied on my relationship with Jesus Christ to help me recover. I finally came to the point where I had to acknowledge my illness and recognize the truth that I would never be able to recover on my own without letting go and trusting Christ in a manner I had not done in the past. The boiling point came after the most painful screaming match I ever had with my husband. It was at that critical point that I realized that I had no strength left—no strength to be angry, no strength to be afraid, no strength to deny my depression any longer. Several days later, after much prayer, I finally discussed my depression with my husband.

> Trusting, truly trusting in a higher power gave me a tremendous sense of optimism and a positive attitude, which I feel is essential to developing the resiliency necessary in fighting a debilitating condition.

ILANA
AT-HOME MOM
MICHIGAN, USA

Taking care of diapering and other physical needs was easy enough. When he cried, though, I didn't know what to do. These were the hardest times. I'd get nervous and upset, question my own abilities, and end up crying myself. I felt guilty that I wasn't doing things right. I was afraid that he'd pick up bad signals from me and get upset.

Later on in my depression, about five months postpartum, I was terrified by my own thoughts. I feared hurting him. I was angry, and I felt guilty about my own anger. I feared I was going crazy, but I was afraid to say anything because I feared my baby would be taken away from me. I didn't like being alone because I thought about suicide and dying in general. It was terrifying!

I was never hospitalized, but during my most painful moments,

I wished for it. My husband and I did discuss admitting me, but fear and finances held us back. I sought outpatient treatment at a Christian mental health facility. The psychiatrist prescribed an antidepressant and also helped me correct my "self-talk" to be more positive. He had me ask myself (when I caught myself putting myself down) if I would say this same thing to a friend. If you wouldn't say it to a friend, then it's best you not say it to yourself. I had to work on becoming less emotive and more realistic. I usually have an urge to go-go-go. I've had to learn that my worth is not measured by my ability to do, accomplish, or succeed. My worth is found in being a beloved creation of God. So I concentrated on "being," instead of "doing."

Now That I've Recovered

Now I feel that being a homemaker is indeed my calling. I never want to go back to the working world. I've been entertaining family and expanding my network of friends. I feel so much more social. My belief in a personal, loving God has helped me hang on when I had feelings of nothing but hopelessness. I had faith that He was always with me, even when my body and mind were telling me I was alone. God is the most reliable part of my support system.

NELLY
24, AT-HOME MOM
TEXAS, USA

The moment my son was put in my arms I didn't feel that instant bond I'd heard women talk about. I fed him, changed him, held him, and played with him, but I felt like a robot. It all seemed mechanical. It was strange because I knew I loved him more than my own life. I just couldn't feel it.

Once the PPD worsened, there were days I couldn't even hold him. The sound of his cry made me sob. I had planned to be a stay-at-home mother, but after seven months it got so bad that we put him in day care three days a week. My husband had two days off, so that left me only two days to care for him. Sometimes I still couldn't handle even that and my husband had to come home from work. That made me beat myself up even more.

I had never experienced insomnia—now I couldn't sleep. My to-do list would flood through my head. When I thought about what I needed to do in a week, I'd become completely immobile. On a good day, I could do a load of laundry. On a bad day, I couldn't even brush my hair. When I awoke, I immediately started to count down the minutes until the end of the day. I couldn't wait to put the baby to bed. As far gone as I was, I still treasured those hours I was alone with my husband.

I felt a million miles away from him and my baby. My husband and I were always so close—best friends. Suddenly I was questioning my marriage and my love. That's what almost pushed me over the edge. Everything felt wrong all the time. I became very clingy around my husband. I wanted to be with him twenty-four hours a day. It was like I was trying to get the feeling back that I thought I'd lost. I knew he felt smothered, but I couldn't help it. If my husband couldn't find someone to cover for him at work, then I'd take the baby to his store, sit, and cry, and he'd take care of both of us between customers.

The scariest parts of PPD were the times I had thoughts of hurting my baby. I had visions of stabbing or smothering him. It was my own private hell. I knew in my heart I'd never do these things, but still, the other part of my mind reasoned that people just like me did snap. If they could lose it, what could prevent me from ending up the same way? I began to have suicidal thoughts: *Perhaps my husband and son would be better off without me.*

I did not have a doctor because right after the baby was born we moved to a new state to be closer to my husband's family. So I went to a walk-in clinic for help. After several tries and bad results with medications, I went to a medical professional who prescribed an antidepressant. I started to feel better in one week. The guilt, depression, and scary thoughts all started to subside. The medication was the miracle that allowed me to be at a level where I could cope and start to heal. I began to look forward to my time alone with my son. One day when I picked him up from day care, he put his arms around my neck and burrowed his head in my chest with a big hug. I knew in that minute that even though he was in day care, he wouldn't forget who I was. I knew I had done the right thing by putting him in day care to allow myself to heal.

My husband was the most important person in my recovery. He constantly reassured me and listened to my problems and sobbing. He had his own problems, but didn't tell me because he knew I wasn't strong enough yet to handle them. If I had to do it over, I would have gotten therapy much sooner, to take the burden off of him.

As the medication kicked in, I would waken in the morning and actually look forward to the day. I hadn't felt that way in a long time. My husband and I finally had a heart-to-heart talk about what we'd been going through. He cried, told me how he just wanted his best friend back. I realized that for him to open up to me, he had to believe I wasn't as fragile anymore. I was recovering. Now I could listen to him, give back emotionally, and not just take.

Now That I've Recovered

I actually enjoy my time with my son. We often take day trips while my husband is working. I know I'm a survivor. I've been to hell and fought my way out. There is nothing life can throw at me that can be worse than the fear of hurting my child. There is nothing scarier than wondering if I might snap and take my own life.

I've learned that I do not need to be perfect at everything I do. To be perfect is to be inhuman. I've learned to just be me—that's who my baby loves, that's who my husband loves, and now that's who I love!

> What lies before us are small matters compared to what lies within us.
>
> —*Ralph Waldo Emerson*

Thoughts for a Better Day

At first, I perceived myself as terribly weak because I got PPD, but I see things so differently now. I don't believe I could have survived it without my inner strength. I focus on living a happy life now. I accept every day as a gift, not as an inevitability to be endured.

Mostly, I have been humbled by the realization that we all have limits. We need help sometimes in our lives and we must ask for it. I am now raising a beautiful, intelligent, and happy son. I am a good wife and friend. I am much stronger than I ever thought I was.

—Sophie, 28, At-Home Mom
Arizona, USA

PEARL
32, PART-TIME ATTORNEY/HOMEMAKER
CALIFORNIA, USA

My expectation about motherhood was that I could work from home with an infant. I didn't think my schedule would change that much. I thought the baby would need me to feed him and change him and he would sleep in his crib or play in his playpen. I didn't think he would cry so much. I didn't realize I would feel so tired after getting up several times to feed him.

My PPD began just days after giving birth and lasted almost eighteen months. I wanted to sleep all the time. I returned to bed as often as I could, and became completely uninterested in sex. My breasts were "off limits" to my husband since the baby needed them. Not only did I become oblivious to my own needs, but I also ignored my husband's needs while trying to satisfy the baby's needs.

I didn't fall instantly in love with my son. I had thoughts of "sending him back," secretly hoping he would die in his sleep so I would not have to face another day of breast-feeding, changing diapers, and feeling guilty. I felt so alone. How could other women say having children was the best thing that ever happened when I felt so horrible?

I cried all the time and didn't know how I could last another day, let alone a month or a year. I didn't want to run errands because I was so lethargic and exhausted. It was such a hassle to get my baby ready to go anywhere. I felt as if I were a prisoner in my own home.

When I confessed my "bad thoughts" about harming the baby to my husband, he professed his love to me and encouraged me, and told me I was doing a great job as a mommy. I received help from a psychologist. Don't wait until you hit rock bottom before you seek help. Learn to open up to people who can help. Many other mothers have similar feelings and troubles. You are struggling with motherhood. You are human.

Thoughts for a Better Day

I had very vivid images of hurting my baby come unbidden to my brain. They weren't something I brought up. It wasn't like, "Oh that brat, I want to kill him" or Velcro him to the wall. That would be a conscious thought process. This was about horrid images just popping into my brain—things I would never think of on my own.

It sounds like I'm splitting hairs, but there is a huge difference. I don't think I would have understood or believed me either, if I hadn't "been there." Unfortunately, I understand what Andrea Yates was doing and how it made "sense" to her to drown her children and how it seemed like her only choice, even if she knew it was wrong. Moms having PPD during Andrea Yates's arrest and trial must have been extremely scared from the fear Andrea's behavior would become their own. It is terrifying to think that perhaps it could have been me.

—Ruth, 46, At-Home Mom
Hawaii, USA

◦◦◦ SAMANTHA ◦◦◦
29, AT-HOME MOM
ONTARIO, CANADA

Now that I've recovered, I have a great home, a happy baby, and a great relationship with my husband. Through the PPD we had to learn to be open to one another, to say everything, and accept each other. Force yourself to get up and go out. Even if you only go out once a week at first and then more often, it will help you to stop thinking about your personal problems. Go at your own rhythm.

Take one day at a time and when it gets to be too much take one minute at a time. Don't forget that one day you'll look back on all of it and say, "I went through it all!"

CHAPTER 4

Mothers with Challenging Childbirths

The most profound experience of any woman's life is the birth of a child. There is probably no other experience more highly anticipated . . . filled with emotion, expectation, wonder, and awe. Women love to share their birth experiences with each other. How long was labor? Was it an easy or a difficult delivery? What is the most memorable part of this miraculous, glorious experience?

For the mothers in Chapter Four, their birth experiences were painful. Mothers with difficult childbirths may experience symptoms of post-traumatic stress disorder, according to Postpartum Support International. PTSD involves long-standing symptoms that follow trauma and can occur from a traumatic labor and delivery.

These birth experiences may have contributed to postpartum depression. A mother from Chapter Four explains it brilliantly: "Labor is a set of contractions . . . and then a mother is born."

~ UMA ~
32, AT-HOME MOM
ENGLAND, U.K.

Our son was born with the umbilical cord pulled tight around his body and twice around his neck. While I was pushing, it was acting like a noose. He was not able to breathe at childbirth, and it took the doctor four full minutes to resuscitate him. The doctors said we were extremely lucky.

It was an hour before I could see him and I was hysterical. I already knew the huge demands of a newborn with my first child at home, but I realize now that the incident and childbirth knocked me for a loop. I was worried that something could go wrong with him. I became overwhelmed with worry for him . . . would he have brain damage, or SIDS, etc. Other than a bout of bronchitis at eight months, he had no other health problems. But *I* was falling into postpartum depression.

At ten weeks postpartum, I was diagnosed. I spent most of my time crying, and withdrew from everyone. Sometimes I couldn't even face my own parents. I felt like I was on autopilot, taking care of my baby. I didn't feel any love for him until he was ten months old. Once I confided to my husband and doctor that I had feared losing control and harming my baby and myself. My doctor wanted to hospitalize me, but I begged them to let me stay home. I was not allowed to be alone with the kids, so I was always under the watchful eye of my husband, parents, aunt, or friends.

My former best friend told me to "Take a couple of pills and snap out of it." I received help from my health visitor, psychiatric nurse, and general practitioner and various antidepressants were prescribed until we found the one that worked for me. My turning points came when I finally realized that I did love my baby and when professional child care at nighttime arrived so I could finally sleep. My

health visitor always told me that there was light at the end of the
tunnel no matter how long this might take. He was quite right!

Now That I've Recovered

> Rejoice in the Lord always, and
> again I say. Rejoice. Let your
> moderation be known unto all
> men. The Lord is at hand. Be
> careful for nothing, but in every-
> thing by prayer and supplication
> with thanksgiving let your re-
> quest be made known unto God.
> —*Phillipians 4:4–6*

Remember, you will make
progress as time goes by, although it may be slow. If you
have understanding friends, talk
to them. They may be able to
help just by listening. Most of
all, remember that you are not
alone. I know lots of mothers at
my children's school who, once
we got talking, said they suffered
the same as I did. Your baby
needs you. Don't try to do things because of social pressure—just
do what you feel is right for you and your baby.

ᴬ Ava ᴬ

32, At-Home Mom
New South Wales, Australia

The whole process of labor and delivery left me feeling violated,
ugly, ashamed, and abused. I was embarrassed about screaming
through the final stages of the delivery, and my throat was parched
and sore. Why were all the other new mothers in the maternity ward
walking around as if they were completely untouched by the act of
having a baby? I felt physically and mentally ill after childbirth. I
could not stop thinking about the agony, as if my tortured body had
been ripped in half. No one seemed to think it was a big deal at all.

Having been a teacher of mathematical and computer studies

for seven years, I considered myself a perfectionist and had high expectations of myself and others. I am organized and like to be in control of my life. But I've since learned that motherhood requires a rapid and thorough change of attitude. Nothing was predictable anymore—except that my baby would cry and I would be sleep deprived.

The ironing piled up, the floors got dirty, and my husband learned to heat up a can of spaghetti. People tell mothers that baby care is easy. Then they ask you why you're not coping. Somehow I thought I would breeze through all of this. Why do mothers have to pretend that their mental health is not going to be affected by massive, rapid change combined with prolonged sleep deprivation? Why can't society support new mothers? Why does PPD have a certain shame attached to it when, in fact, it is the most logical manifestation on the face of the earth?

After I breast-fed, I barely had the energy to button up my blouse. I could not comprehend how other new mothers could be going out to lunch. I wondered if I could get out of the chair. I checked myself into a two-night stay at a hospital due to exhaustion. I was given sleeping tablets and asked whether I wanted to see a counselor. I declined, still not knowing I had PPD, but I was nearing a state of crisis. My mood swings were getting worse. I decided to move me and my baby to my parents' home, where we sought help for six weeks. It was our family doctor who finally diagnosed me with PPD. Putting a name to my misery gave me relief and hope. I did not elect to take the recommended antidepressants, and ultimately, nature, time, and patience were my "physicians."

Thoughts for a Better Day

Look upon your PPD experience as a time of great personal growth. It is the most common illness that affects women after childbirth. When you recover, you will finally enjoy your baby.

> Perfect love casteth out fear be-
> cause fear hath torment.
>
> —John 4:18

Once you admit to others you had PPD, you'll find it amazing to hear other mothers admit the troubles they endured during those frantic newborn days. You are not alone. All over the world, the proverbial wheel is being reinvented as mothers and fathers struggle through those difficult days. As a friend of mine put it, "Labor is a set of contractions . . . and then a mother is born."

⟶ STEVIE ⟵
28, AT-HOME MOM
UTAH, USA

During the whole twenty-seven-hour delivery and recovery I was surprised by the difference the nurses could make to my attitude. I had two nurses who were so negative about the state of my baby's health, before and after delivery, that I stayed awake worrying both nights I was in the hospital. In contrast, there were nurses who were reassuring about the normalcy of a few setbacks to the baby during a long, hard labor. Unfortunately, I spoke to these nurses after I had spent the night stewing.

Thoughts for a Better Day

I'm the kind of person who always looked at others with emotional problems and thought they just lacked self-control. How grateful I am that my family didn't feel the same about me! They never stopped trying to get me to look at the positive side or to get up and do something to take my mind off it. But they did not accuse me of wallowing in self-pity. Now that I've been to the other side of a psychological disorder, I have a great sympathy for others who suffer from them. PPD is not a weakness—it is a disease. You deserve help. Demand it! It's not fair, but it's not permanent!

⤙ EYDIE ⤚
32, DEAN OF STUDENT SERVICES
CALIFORNIA, USA

The pushing process was horrendous for me. My body was shaking so hard and uncontrollably and my teeth were chattering. When her head popped out, I screamed bloody murder at the top of my lungs—and then the shoulders came out. I thought I was going to die. The whole birthing process shook me to the core. I told the nurse not to let go of my daughter when she brought her to me because I was too weak to hold her.

Thoughts for a New Day

All I ever heard about were women who were so happy staying home with their babies. That's great for them, but I had to eventually accept that it wasn't for me. I was raised to be independent and ambitious—not to depend on a man for happiness, so I've worked hard to conquer my guilt about being "happy" not being a stay-at-home mom. I've adjusted nicely now to my role as mother and a working woman again.

⤙ HANNAH ⤚
26, AT-HOME MOM
ONTARIO, CANADA

Intellectually I know a smooth delivery doesn't always happen . . . but in my heart it just never occurred to me that I'd need a C-section.

While I was thankful to deliver a healthy baby boy, I felt empty and cheated of the chance to push my son out into the world as nature had intended, with my husband at my side.

Then my baby had trouble breast-feeding and he was losing weight. He was colicky for seven months and I grew more and more depressed and angry with a baby who hated to be cuddled, and refused to be consoled by me. The only time he ever wanted me was when he was hungry.

The possibility of PPD never even occurred to me. Although I'd heard of it, the wretched feelings of despair and self-loathing I was experiencing were, I assumed, just manifestations of my inadequacy as a mother. I was a horrible person, a dud mom, and that was that. Feeding, bathing, and changing my son brought me no joy—just misery. I was wracked with deep guilt as I put on a phony smile and told people I loved motherhood.

I was nervous, irritable, and unable to sleep or nap when my son napped. I had manic insomnia. Lack of sleep took its toll on me— my sobbing and mood swings became more and more severe. By about three months postpartum, I was eyeing the kitchen knives and imagining hurting myself. I wanted to run off into the night and curl up in a ball and die. My family physician suggested I take antidepressants, but I still didn't believe I had PPD, just a series of circumstances that were responsible for my emotional state. I thought it would be selfish of me to take the drugs because I'd have to stop breast-feeding. So he dropped the subject, but urged me to call if I felt even the slightest impulse to harm myself or my son.

That moment came one month later when, after listening to my son scream for an hour, I grabbed him, held him up to my face, and screamed right back at him. Shock and fear appeared on his face— I'm still deeply ashamed. I hugged and kissed him while sobbing and calling my doctor. After trying several medications, I found the one that helped. Within two weeks I felt better than I had since my son's birth. I could finally get through the day without shedding a single tear. Soon I could breathe deeply, smile sincerely, and feel loving and maternal to my baby. I remained on medication for nine months.

Now That I've Recovered

I've since had two more children and two even stronger cases of PPD. I must continue on the medication every day, but I've learned that taking medication enables me to cope. I'm simply a victim of what I jokingly refer to as "stupid brain chemistry." Taking medication is the mature and loving thing to do for my family.

> Making the decision to have a child—it's momentous. It is to decide forever to have your heart go walking outside your body.
>
> —Elizabeth Stone

⟡ SUELLYN ⟡
38, REGISTERED NURSE
ALBERTA, CANADA

After seven hours of labor at home with my midwife, we went to the hospital as planned. Then *wham-bam*, everything happened. Too many people were talking to me, too much excitement, and all I remember was a terrifying voice saying, "We have to get this baby out now!"

I later learned that they had lost my baby's heartbeat. I had an emergency C-section with general anesthesia, and delivered a flat, floppy baby girl with an Apgar of 1 (she had a bit of a heartbeat and that was all). They kept her in a special-care nursery for twenty-four hours. I just wanted them to give her to me—it was awful.

PPD hit me right away and lasted about one year. I was very emotional and had many crying spells. The more exhausted I became, the more I withdrew from family and friends. I suffered from panic attacks. A girlfriend of mine had experienced postpartum psychosis and referred me to a gentle, kind therapist. She asked me what was the one thing that bothered me the most about my birth experience and, although my head was full of so many thoughts, I replied, "I didn't get to see my daughter right away. I wasn't there for her when she came out. Everyone got to see her before me."

My therapist was a very spiritual woman, and she probed further. She wanted to know what it was like when my daughter was born. I told her I was too out of it to know. I was under general anesthesia for the emergency C-section, but she gently asked, "What was your daughter like when she was born?" And I told her that she was flat, floppy, almost dead, not breathing. She told me, "You were in the right place—you went to go get her. You brought her back to this world."

She believed that because I was not in this world, not in my conscious state, that I was able to go to bring my daughter out of her near death—so I had "been there" for my daughter the whole time. As crazy as it may sound, it was the one thing that really worked for me. The therapist reframed my birth experience. She invited me to consider the possibility that my daughter and I (both being other-worldly at the time) were together at birth. My spirit went to join her spirit and we came back together. Now I could see what was good about this birth. After feeling so incredibly bummed for so long, this realization helped me "turn the corner" to recovery.

> Stores have handicapped parking but I believe they ought to have "postpartum parking" for brand-new mothers trying to hobble their pain-stricken bodies and babies into the store to pick up a jug of milk, diapers, or whatever they need.
>
> —Jordanna, 23, Student Teacher
> New Mexico, USA

CHAPTER 5

Mothers with
Breast-Feeding Issues

Most women believe that breast-feeding is a natural step to becoming a new mother . . . nature provides us with all we need to nourish our babies. Women look forward to the amazing bond that is formed with our infant through this seemingly natural process.

So when problems arrive with breast-feeding—if the baby doesn't latch on, or if there is not enough milk, or if there is pain—mothers may experience a great sense of anxiety or loss. A mother may feel inadequate. She has put so much pressure on herself to breast-feed for the sake of the baby . . . and yet she may be unable to achieve those expectations.

There is plenty of pressure from breast-feeding organizations for mothers to nurse their babies. But mothers who are facing breast-feeding difficulties should not be faced with a guilt trip if they need to quit or choose bottle feeding. Like the previous chapter of experiences of mothers with difficult deliveries, these mothers who experienced breast-feeding difficulties may have been more likely to develop postpartum depression.

～❧ HAZEL ❧～
32, TEACHER
NORTH CAROLINA, USA

I planned to breast-feed my daughter, but when my milk came in, my breasts became engorged and my milk wouldn't let down. I had no idea what went wrong and I thought I had failed in some way. Three days after birth at the doctor checkup, my daughter had lost weight. As new parents, we were so scared. Although a lactation consultant helped us, it became so traumatic to breast-feed that I began supplementing with formula.

I became very anxious, tense, and upset when I nursed her. I felt selfish and guilty for feeling so sad. I thought I was supposed to be "glowing" in the light of motherhood. I had had two previous bouts of depression in my life, but nothing compared to the despair I felt postpartum.

When I got pregnant, I had just finished my master's degree and my sixth year of teaching. I had no idea how physically and emotionally difficult new motherhood would be. I love working with children as a teacher and I adore my nieces and nephews. Everyone always commented, "You'll be such a good mother." My sister made motherhood look so easy. It wasn't until after I told her my feelings that she told me she had felt the same way. I guess people just don't talk about it. I had read some articles about PPD, and I thought I might be affected because of my history. But nothing prepared me for what it was really like. Talking with my sister helped me to not feel so alone.

Recovery was a slow process. My medical professional prescribed an antidepressant and I started to feel better six weeks later. I joined a PPD support group and connected with a mother there. We shared honestly about how things were going, and it was a huge support. At five and a half weeks postpartum, I took my daughter out for the first time alone. I met my friend at the mall for pizza. We started a new "Mommy & Me" group with a dozen moms and babies that helped so much. And I went to work after maternity leave. I knew how to be a good teacher and I found instant gratification.

Thoughts for a Better Day

My biggest accomplishment *is* recovering from PPD. It amazes me every day how at ease I feel with my daughter now. I'm able to feel such joy now when I look at her, rather than the fear and sadness I originally felt. Experiencing PPD has made me appreciate every day when I wake up happy and able to be the mother

> Each child carries his own blessing into the world.
> —*Yiddish proverb*

I want to be. My daughter is nearly a year old now and I can't imagine my life without her. She brings us such happiness.

Remember, it's okay not to be in love with your baby the moment you see that new life arrive. At first you're strangers. In time, when PPD passes, you'll love your child at depths you could never have imagined.

～ GRACE ～
32, CHARITY FUND-RAISER
ENGLAND, U.K.

My overwhelming feeling upon my son's birth was a sense of relief that he was out and safe and the belief that things could only get better. Ha! Breast-feeding was an agonizing and deeply unpleasant experience. After developing mastitis and a breast abscess, I gave up breast-feeding at two weeks postpartum. I remember sobbing in my mother's arms (something I've not ever done as an adult) and telling her I couldn't cope.

It was the first time I realized that I really wasn't well. I'm usually a very independent person who performs well under pressure. The next day I felt as if I were drowning when I read the congratulations cards and messages of support. It seemed everyone was overjoyed at my son's arrival—except for me. I felt alone and mean for not being overjoyed. After wanting a baby so much, now all I could do was wallow in misery.

People I'm close to have all said that, from my behavior, they would never have guessed that I had PPD. At face value, I was as loving toward him as a tired mum can be. I made every effort to interact and bond. Inside, however, I felt like a fake, just going through the motions, making the right "cooing" and comfort noises because I knew how, not because I wanted to. I remember a friend describe to me how she would watch her son sleeping, wishing secretly that he would wake up so that she could play with him. This seemed like such an alien desire. I thought with envy how wonderful it must be to be relaxed enough to feel that way. Thank goodness there was great bonding going on between my son and his father.

> Always know how important you are as a parent. God has allowed for you to be the channel for another one of his precious souls to enter the world.
>
> —Unknown

My baby dictated when I could sleep, eat, talk, walk . . . everything. I was at his beck and call. I could neither live with him nor without him. He was the center of my world, but I was resistant to sharing with him. He sapped my energy and yet gave energy to me to somehow survive—a very fragile balance that I fought to gain control over.

The health visitor told me to stop worrying about things that might not ever happen, and that was exactly what I needed to do—

only I didn't know how. I just couldn't let go of my fears, and I became overprotective of my son. I never felt suicidal, but for the first time in my life I felt I really understood how thin the line is between good and ill mental health. My health visitor finally convinced me (I had resisted) to see a doctor, and an antidepressant was prescribed. A month later I felt calm and in control. I stayed on it eight months. My son began going to my parents three days each week and I started to catch up on rest. Gradually I became fit again and remembered who I was.

Now That I've Recovered

I am now better equipped to cope with any bouts of depression. I have the confidence to say it will not go on forever; I will get better. This is the most important thing to remember. To experience the highs in life, you have to be able to understand the lows.

⇁ Mariah ⇀
32, At-Home Mom
Texas, USA

I expected my baby to latch on and suck, but instead he screamed. He seemed to hate it. We were discharged less than twenty-four hours after birth. I didn't want to go home. I felt so weak. I spent the next three days in the house with no help (my mom only stayed a day or two), and I tried to breast-feed every two hours. Instead I listened to a screaming baby.

The isolation and loneliness was devastating. It is so overwhelming being in charge of this little life twenty-four hours a day. I couldn't rest. After trying for a week and working with lactation consultants, I was so miserable I quit breast-feeding. I have regretted that decision ever since. I called the lactation consultant back when my son was three months old to see about breast-feeding again, but she said it would be very difficult, with no guarantee I'd produce enough milk.

I attribute a great deal of my PPD to my breast-feeding failure. I felt sad, cheated, and bitter that I didn't experience the wonderful nursing relationship that the books I read talked about. He was colicky, too, and I had intense anger at God for allowing a baby to cry so much. He was a poor sleeper and because I needed sleep so bad I was also angry that God gave me a son I obviously couldn't handle. I was physically and emotionally exhausted and didn't think I had patience for a demanding infant.

I wore myself out reading books on crying babies as I tried to figure out why he was so unhappy. I never let him cry himself to sleep, as I didn't think that would work. I withdrew from anyone who was a "happy" mommy. At six weeks postpartum, I saw my psychiatrist who I knew from a previous bout with depression. He prescribed antidepressants.

> God doesn't call on us to be successful; he calls on us to be faithful.
>
> —Mother Teresa

At one year postpartum, I stupidly decided it was time to be over this and quit my medication. I had a really bad day . . . of wanting to be locked up or die. I got right back on my medication and began to feel better again. Time was the big healer. I started going to play groups and made new mommy friends. I felt more in control of my life, but it was a slow healing process.

Now That I've Recovered

The ordeal was so painful that I remember thinking my son would be an only child because I wouldn't risk going through PPD again. But the pain healed, and I did have a second child, and I did endure PPD again.

Now I have a much stronger faith in God. As a result of these depressions I started going to church and I've become much more understanding of others with mental illnesses. I don't think I judge people the way I used to do.

⤜ OLIVIA ⤛
34, BANQUET SERVER
WASHINGTON, USA

With mastitis it hurt so much to breast-feed, but I knew the benefits of breast-feeding and I was committed to it. My mother said I should just give my baby a bottle so I could get some relief. But I think the breast-feedings saved us. It kept my daughter and me connected and helped me stay in love with her, despite my PPD.

My mother came into town for the birth but went right back home after the hospital stay because she wanted us "to have time to bond as a family." I live in a very remote area. The sleep deprivation was taking its toll and I knew I was in the middle of PPD after I read an entry in a book about a woman who had it. On one particular night she thought about putting her baby outside. If her baby survived the night, she'd bring her back in, but if not, she figured it wasn't meant to be. I could actually relate to these scary thoughts.

Two friends who knew I had PPD came to stay with me and help—they ascended like angels. A First Steps area counselor became my friend and she would stop by and monitor my baby and me. This made a huge difference. I would think, "How many days until she comes again? Oh good, I can make it till then." She gave me hope.

My turning point came with the spring (my baby was born in December), and with simply getting past the infant stage—which scared me to death. When she was six months old, I started a PPD support group. Sharing stories with other new mothers greatly helped my transition into parenthood.

Now That I've Recovered

We can never know what to expect as new mothers, but we must remain open—not get attached to a certain outcome. We need to let the mystery in. Leave room for the unexpected; count on it. If I had only known this, it would have been a lot easier.

QUINTA
33, COMPUTER TECHNICIAN
CONNECTICUT, USA

I tried to breast-feed for the first three weeks, however, because my daughter was premature, she lost weight during the first week, which caused concern from the doctor. I remember a particularly unsupportive nurse at the hospital, who told me that my daughter had lost weight and had to be put under a heat lamp because her temperature had dropped, and then asked me if those "lactation people" had told me to stop giving my daughter formula. I then became obsessed with her weight and not being able to measure the amount of breast milk she received made me very nervous. I switched to formula—my pediatrician supported the decision—however, I still felt a tremendous guilt for stopping the breast-feeding.

Everyone tells you that once you have a child, your life is never the same, but I didn't comprehend what that meant. I was not prepared to lose my independence for this new person who depended on me for everything. I also thought there was this wonderful thing called maternal instinct, that I'd know how to soothe my baby's cries. I discovered I hadn't the slightest clue as to what to do. The childbirth classes spent so much time talking about the birth (which

I ended up having no control over anyway), and very little time talking about taking care of the baby. I felt totally unprepared.

I resented my husband, too. I was jealous that he got to go to work and get on with his life, and I was home. I was miserable and wanted him to be just as miserable. My husband was the only one who knew I was depressed (my mother had always given me the impression that asking for help was a sign of weakness), and he urged me to get help. But I thought if I could just get one good night's sleep—and if he helped out more—I'd be okay.

But I was totally focused on how much I hated being a mother. I wanted to use my arms for something other than holding and rocking. I felt like a household drudge, caught in the monotony of feeding, burping, and changing this crying, demanding stranger. Everyone else seemed to enjoy mother-hood, but I was bored, frustrated, and lonely. When my daughter cried her colicky cries, my only peace was to leave her in her crib and take a shower. It drowned out her cries and no one could hear mine.

> Don't worry about the mess in your home. Don't expect to be super-mom. If you have clean underwear and the baby has clean clothes, you are doing great!
> —Carmen, Administrative Assistant
> Winnipeg, Canada

I felt there was something wrong with me, but I didn't yet realize what it was. When my daughter was six months old, I pulled into the garage after she spent the entire ride howling in the backseat. I laid my head on the steering wheel, cried, and seriously contemplated clicking the button to let the garage door close behind us. Luckily thoughts of my husband made me turn off the car. The next day I made an appointment with a psychiatrist who specialized in PPD.

An antidepressant was prescribed for me. It took a month to feel better, and I stayed on it for six months. I think the medication just lifted a huge cloud from me. I didn't realize what a fog I was living in until it was gone. The little things didn't bother me and the crying stopped. I felt like I could actually breathe again.

Now That I've Recovered

My husband and I get along much better now and I enjoy every minute I spend with our daughter. I marvel at her accomplishments.

Remember, it's okay to be sad, but you don't have to be sad forever. Get help in any way that works for you. Ask for and accept help. I found that seeing a third party was less stressful than help from well-meaning family members.

CHAPTER 6

Mothers with Ill Babies

Every mother hopes and prays to deliver a healthy baby. We are overjoyed when we hear that first cry after baby's first breath. But for mothers who deliver a premature or ill baby, delivery becomes traumatizing. The anxiety over the baby's well-being, and the worry about what the future holds, add significant stress to postpartum adjustment. These feelings and worries can lead mothers to develop postpartum depression as described here in Chapter Six.

~❦~ GABRIELLA ~❦~
31, AT-HOME MOM
MASSACHUSETTS, USA

My daughter was born at only thirty-two weeks gestation, weighing just over two pounds. Because she was premature, she was in NICU for sixty days. Although she was too weak to breast-feed, I pumped my breasts for six months so she could receive breast milk.

When she finally came home, I had a hard time bonding with her. I believe that I knew what to expect with the physical demands of being a mother because for the past nine years I was an R.N. in the maternity ward. But I did not expect the emotional demands. Nobody understood this when I voiced that feeling. It was very isolating. Ironically, as a nurse I used to educate new mothers about postpartum depression. And now I was the one worried because I believed that if a child doesn't feel an emotional bond, that child might not learn or trust, which is important in development.

I often experience feelings of guilt now because I wasn't there for her emotionally at the beginning. During my fourteen months with PPD, I did not have sleep problems. And I don't think I was highly irritable and emotional. If anything, I was quite the opposite: detached, numb, and lethargic, not motivated to do anything I used to enjoy, including running. After trying to discuss my feelings with my husband and mother, I realized they seemed horrified by what I told them, so I withdrew.

I never lacked confidence in my ability to physically care for my baby, but it was more as if I wasn't there for her emotionally. Everything seemed cloudy and overwhelming. I never sought professional help or any medication. A turning point came when I interviewed and was hired for a part-time job. I realized that I would have to leave my daughter with my mother and aunt two days a week, and I didn't want to leave her for even that amount of time! I knew then I had bonded with her. Also, when I told one of my old friends that I was having a hard time bonding with my daughter, she confided in me that she also experienced those feelings with her second child. It was such a relief to have someone understand. Isolation is such an enemy.

Now That I've Recovered

This month, I am involved in a charity walk for the March of Dimes, to support a cause that contributed to my daughter's health. The March of Dimes was responsible for funding the development of a medication given to me prior to my child's birth to mature her lungs.

When you are faced with adversity, sometimes your first reaction is to just run away, but you become stronger with each little battle you win, and then slowly you realize that you have won the war over your personal demons. It's a process, and it has made me a much more empathetic and genuine person.

> Obstacles are those frightful things you see when you take your eyes off the goal.
>
> —Henry Ford

✑ DANIELLE ✑
30, CLERK
NEW SOUTH WALES, AUSTRALIA

After two weeks of great difficulty breast-feeding, our son was checked for and diagnosed with a urinary tract infection. He was hospitalized for a week. Throughout the ordeal, we found great difficulty in getting medical staff to listen to us when we described what was wrong with him. After returning home from the hospital, I put him on a formula and he has thrived ever since.

My mother was the first to actually suspect that I had a problem. She said something wasn't right with me five days after childbirth. After seven weeks she confronted me with her concern. My main symptom was that I cried every day for four months. A good day was just one cry session. But sometimes they happened all day long—hours and hours. My eyes were red and swollen as if someone had hit me. I often wondered if you could run out of tears. Apparently not.

I had days when I couldn't be left alone to cope. My family took turns staying with me for company. They didn't actually do anything to help care for the baby, but I needed someone to be with me "just in case." In case of what, I'm not really sure. I was very emotional, but not very irritable. I couldn't get my head around any other feeling but total, utter sadness. I was in a fog. Like my head was full of cotton wool or cotton candy. I just floated around and didn't act much like myself.

I also felt like there was a big, black, gaping crack in my chest that widened to a point you could see right inside of me to my breaking heart. I had a lot of problems with invasive thoughts. The main one was "You were infertile for a reason. You should never have had children." This still nearly brings me to tears to even think it. I have polycystic ovary syndrome and I think the fertility drugs contributed greatly to my depression. I saw my general practitioner, then a community psychologist, and finally a psychiatrist who specialized in PPD. He was fantastic—knew exactly the right questions to ask. He changed my antidepressant and the relief was amazing. My husband and family provided great support, but the medication was the savior here. I had no way of lifting myself out of the tar pit without it. It gave me relief to think like myself again and get on with my normal life. My husband has said often that he is so glad I am "back" now.

Thoughts for a Better Day

If you have PPD, try to believe it will get better. Hug your baby close at least once a day, actually telling him you love him. No matter how much it hurts you and you think the pain will never stop, the baby needs you and you need him. Get help. I cannot stress this enough. There is a light at the end of the tunnel—you just don't know how long the tunnel will be.

Thoughts for a Better Day

You are doing the most important thing in the world—parenting. There is no other "job" that is more respected, understood, and worthwhile than this. Think of yourself as being truly blessed if you are given the gift of raising a child. This is true even if your child is born with birth defects. These defects will soon prove not to be deficits but rather attributes, so celebrate throughout your child's life.

Get a headset telephone. This will allow you to talk to friends, your mom, or your doctor while holding the baby and doing chores.

—Jordanna, 23, Teacher
New Mexico, USA

CHAPTER 7

Mothers with Colicky Babies

New mothers are keenly attuned to their babies' cries. Their first concern is to comfort. Mothers with colicky babies endure seemingly endless hours upon hours of hearing their babies cry. Colicky babies will not respond to Mother's urgent attempts to soothe, no matter how hard she tries. As the mothers in Chapter Seven describe, they must simply "ride out" the storms of screaming. For postpartum mothers who suffer from sleep deprivation and exhaustion, a colicky baby contributes to an extra stressful beginning of motherhood.

INGA

34, SINGER
ZURICH, SWITZERLAND

The first few months were a holy living terror. My son would scream for an hour after every feeding and would scream nonstop for two to three hours between six and eleven P.M. He would writhe in pain, completely inconsolable. It broke my heart to see him in such pain and half the time I was crying right along with him. Because I was breast-feeding, I thought it was something I was eating that was bothering him. My husband would always ask me: "What did you eat today?" as if it was my fault! I cut out so many things: cow's milk, beans, chocolate, sugar, carbonated drinks (even bubbly water), you name it. It got to the point where I was eating only bread and drinking water.

When my mother left after staying the first several weeks, I fell into a deeper depression. I wanted desperately to be taken care of myself, but I had this helpless little baby who needed to be taken care of even more than I did. It ripped me apart inside. I was scared to leave home because I was afraid the baby would cry. When he cried, I became so nervous. I didn't want him to feel bad—ever.

My father-in-law would say things like, "It's not so bad," and "All women go through this." He told me for the umpteenth time that crying was good for a baby's lungs. My husband said I should meet other mothers, but I resented his advice. I envied his "freedom" and would pick a fight with him as soon as he walked in the house from work. Men do not have a clue how hard it can be.

Now That I've Recovered

The simplest and most effective thing that helped me was taking a walk every day with my son. It doesn't have to be a long walk—sometimes just to the end of the block. I'm happy to say I've resumed teaching from my home. I have a series of orchestral concerts set up as a soloist. And I am a much nicer wife again.

~ KEIRA ~

32, AT-HOME MOM
NORTH CAROLINA, USA

During the last three months of pregnancy, I gloried in my bulging body. I gained thirty-six pounds and I felt "holy." As I connected with the "little puncher" inside, my prayer life increased, and I began to have a sense of the responsibility that was coming. But looking back, I now think that all the attention pregnant women get is a cruel setup for what comes after the baby is born.

Our baby had milk intolerance and cried almost constantly for eight weeks. During these crying weeks, I felt so fragile. And I felt angry, too. I thought I had made a very big mistake. Of course, I could not tell anyone these thoughts. The days seemed long and dark. I cried all the time. One day when I burped her, I started banging her on the back. I had snapped. That's when I started calling everyone I could think of for help.

I told my husband about my mini-anxiety attacks, my aching jaw from clenching, and how it seemed hard to breathe and swallow sometimes. I felt as if I were in a constant state of "fight or flight." Just the toaster popping would startle me. I told him how happy I was to be away from our baby. He and I went to see a doctor. I was put on thyroid medication for being severely hypothyroid. I felt better for three weeks, but at my next period I came crashing down. I was put on an antidepressant and improved, but was also put on progesterone therapy to prevent extreme PMS with my cycles.

Therapy has been a blessing. Discovering my need for "middle ground" is a challenge, but also a relief. I no longer "do it all," nor do I do it at a pace I used to do it. I've found support through a "mothers' helpers" group, where twelve-year-old helpers baby-sit while I nap in the other room. And my daughter spends at least two hours with her dad on Saturday and Sunday while I rest.

Now That I've Recovered

Our family has pulled together during this trial. I do not regret this incredibly difficult year. I have grown so much on this journey. My husband really stepped up when I was down. I'm involved in our local Mothers Club now, and look forward to weekly playgroups. We've postponed our next pregnancy plans, now that we have a better notion of what to expect when I'm expecting!

NAOMI
29, SALES TRAINER
WEST VIRGINIA, USA

I became depressed about three weeks postpartum. I remember my father-in-law gazing at his new grandson and remarking, "It makes you wonder how anyone could leave a baby on the church doorsteps."

I thought, "I wonder how anyone doesn't leave them on the doorsteps!"

I would knock myself out trying to be a good mom and do the right things, and the baby would only cry more and more and more. Every day was an insult and another indication of my ineptitude. I kept thinking that the reason no one ever tells people about how hard this really is is because nobody would ever have a baby if they knew the truth. I wanted to throw him against the wall when he wouldn't stop crying. He sounded like an engine that wouldn't turn over . . . a dull, "waaaaahhh, waaaahhh," over and over.

I knew I would never harm him, but the feelings that welled up inside did cause me concern. I would get so freaked out because of all the articles that say that babies are sensitive to Mom's mood—well, that must have meant he knew I secretly hated him. No wonder he was crying! It was a horrible cycle.

At the same time, I had an overwhelming feeling of not being good enough. It was as if the house was haunting me: The laundry was moaning; the unmade bed was crying out; the dishes were screaming. I had hallucinations when I nursed my son in the wee hours of the morning, seeing bugs crawling on the walls or across the carpet. I had suicidal thoughts often.

My best friend, who lived in another state, kept telling me to go on medication. She had had PPD after the births of three of her children, so I always knew the reason for my problem. I went to see my OB/GYN at my four-week checkup and after telling all, through my sobs, he told me to simply pump breast milk and get out of the house—go to the mall. I was so numb that I merely nodded.

I walked out of his office and called my mother, still sobbing. I secretly wanted her to call him and tell him what a stupid man he was, but she didn't. Instead, she made an appointment for me with a woman doctor she knew who was also a new mom. My mother told her I had "baby blues." After seeing me, this doctor said this was not baby blues—I was downright depressed. The psychiatrist prescribed an antidepressant and I reconnected with my friend for support. I relied on my husband a lot, too, and attended a weekly breast-feeding support group. While it wasn't a place to talk about PPD, we did talk openly about things going on in our lives, and it helped a lot.

Now That I've Recovered

My motto is: "Better life through chemistry!" Check with your doctor first on what antidepressant you can safely use while breast-feeding. The best thing you can do for your baby is to get better, no matter what. Ask for help. Get to the doctor.

‑✎‑ ERICA ‑✎‑
35, AT-HOME MOM
NEW BRUNSWICK, CANADA

Although he was still premature, my son was completely healthy. But he was colicky. He fussed constantly. I breast-fed for three months. I would have done so longer, but I was so exhausted that my milk supply dried up. I remember when I was pregnant some people would say that after I had the baby I "might cry." I cried every day for hours. I resented my husband. He could "escape" to work every day while I was left with this screaming, smelly alien. And when he came home at night I did housework and domestic chores while he relaxed with a sleeping baby, watched TV, or slept. I used to yell at him every evening.

I am an organization freak and found it extremely hard to cope with all the chaos and confusion of having a house totally out of control. People kept coming to visit, dirty dishes and laundry piled up, there were no groceries, etc. . . . I was so sleep-deprived that I was dead tired all the time.

I hated my baby and had vivid fantasies about killing him. It scared the hell out of me. I felt so completely alone. I would look around the room while trying to calm the screaming baby, and see the dust, the unopened mail, the empty fridge, and resent my baby for taking so much of my time. I spent every minute with him since I was breast-feeding. I never got a break. Just the cat wanting food

> Time is a great healer. I now find it hard to remember everything I felt and you do forget. Nature fixed it that way. I'm still trying to shed the pounds—what's the rush? I'll do it eventually. And like my midwife said—it kept him warm for nine months!
>
> —Bella, 33, Writer/Director
> England, U.K.

would make me feel overwhelmed. I truly regretted having the baby.

When visitors came, I was always unwashed and in a nightgown. I just didn't have the energy to get cleaned up and go out. I was sure I was doing something wrong because the baby cried so much. I felt overweight, out of shape, ugly, dirty, and smelly with leaky boobs and stitches that pulled and burned.

When I went to my doctor she didn't prescribe anything besides, "Get some sleep." Yes, sleep deprivation was the root of all evil. When I started supplementing breast-feeding with formula at about six weeks postpartum, I got to sleep a couple of hours at a time. I started to feel a little less crazy. Eventually my baby began sleeping some in the morning so I could get some "me" time. I started to catch up on housework and get some control back in my life.

Get help with everything any way you can. It does not make you a bad mother if you can't do it all by yourself. It wasn't until I recovered that I opened up—I was amazed to learn that almost every woman I spoke to had the same feelings about harming their babies, hating their husbands, and resenting their loss of freedom. It was very comforting to find this out—I had been ashamed and embarrassed about how I felt. But not anymore.

Eve
27, At-Home Mom
Virginia, USA

She was colicky. In fact, while we were still in the hospital, the nursery nurse gave her back to me in the middle of the night because she wouldn't stop crying. The colic lasted for two months. I thought I had very realistic expectations about motherhood because I had been a nanny while my husband was in law school. But I was totally overwhelmed by the mastitis, colic, and isolation.

I would be housebound all day alone with the baby. Then when my husband came home from school, we'd trade off walking and consoling our colicky baby. We tried too hard to keep up with our old lifestyle and to control everything. I was so set on doing everything the way I saw other moms do it that I didn't take it easy. I lost my appetite. This was so scary. I would look at my full dinner plate and cry at the table.

I remember being unable to laugh at sitcoms on TV. My husband would be laughing, but I didn't have my usual sense of humor. I was worried about caring for my baby. I feared that I would be put in a psych center forever, and my daughter would not have me as her mum. I had an embarrassing and horrible fear that I would sexually molest her. Thank God I never acted it out, but it was bizarre. I also thought my father-in-law would sexually molest her—another irrational fear. Perhaps I was having post-traumatic stress disorder from having been date-raped in my past.

I telephoned the woman who had visited our Baby Steps class and talked about PPD. She referred me to a medical professional who prescribed antidepressants. After just two weeks I started to feel better. And I met another mother with PPD. I recovered with her constant companionship and empathy.

Now That I've Recovered

I am so grateful for the healing medication, the acknowledgment of what I survived from friends and family, and the awareness of PPD today compared to years ago. Just know *you are not alone.* Call the support groups. Don't be afraid of taking medication. I believe it saved my life! You did nothing to deserve this. Take care of yourself. Put your feet up and let the housework go. Don't be ashamed—talk about it because you might just help another woman with it.

CHAPTER 8

Mothers with Multiples

I remember the shock on my doctor's face when I told him how thrilled I'd be to have a multiple childbirth. I'm a twin and enjoyed having a "best friend" while growing up. Also, I was the youngest of six children and wanted to have a large family like the one I grew up in. So once I became pregnant I explained to my doctor how I felt. After all, wouldn't it just be easier to have several babies at once instead of having to endure several pregnancies?

My doctor just rolled his eyes. I suspect because he knew how difficult multiples really are, making pregnancy more risky and motherhood more demanding. I can now appreciate how immensely difficult it must be to mother multiples. Sleep difficulties are compounded. Fears and anxieties are doubled or tripled. The mothers in Chapter Eight are doubly and triply blessed—but that realization and joy only comes after moms have overcome PPD.

~✿ NATALIE ✿~
24, AT-HOME MOM
OHIO, USA

The hospital was wonderful and supportive during this trying time. We brought the twins home when they each weighed three and a half pounds. We had very little help. Friends and family never visited too long. My mom would help with laundry, but she worked full-time, so it wasn't often. I never realized how little sleep a new mother actually gets, especially with twins. My husband worked swing shift and we were both so tired and on edge with each other. I had worked in child care with four or five infants alone—yet having twins was more work and stress than that.

My close friend tried to get me to go out for dinner or shopping, but it was so hard to take them out because they both had reflux. I loved them, but I thought bonding took longer because they were in the hospital, premature, and *I* couldn't nurse them. When we brought them home, I was so tired and busy, I felt like a robot. The girls were so demanding and never napped at the same time. The house was always a mess. The laundry was piled high. The expenses were building. I never took time for myself.

If I got to take a shower and get dressed it was a good day. I felt bad because I didn't feel like playing with the girls. I never felt like hurting them—more like crawling under a rock forever. I connected with a "mothers of twins" group and it was so nice to see other moms going through the same things as me. We shared tips and came up with ways to simplify tasks. I stopped worrying about what other

> A funny thing happened to me during postpartum depression. I discovered my wet laundry in the refrigerator instead of the dryer!
> —Marianne, 36, At-Home Mom
> Ontario, Canada

people told me I should be doing with the girls. When I got dirty looks for taking them out in socks and no shoes I would just smile. The same if they would start crying in a store.

The pediatrician said it was okay for them to take walks, even in cool weather, and it was good for us to get out of the house. I started taking their photos and began a scrapbook—that's when I realized how fast they grow! They are only little once, so you have to endure the sleepless nights, know they will end, and try to make the best of everything.

Now That I've Recovered

I feel much stronger and truly understand what being a mommy is all about. Now whenever I go to a baby shower, I always include a little note in the gift card to tell the soon-to-be mother that I am available to help, or just talk anytime.

❧ JUDY ❧
29, AT-HOME MOM
OHIO, USA

Two days after I gave birth to twins I became depressed. It lasted six months. I was so anxious I became frozen in an almost hyper-vigilant state and could never sleep. I felt totally out of control as a new mom—deeply alone and overwhelmingly responsible, extraordinarily irritable and emotional.

Friends would phone from around the country and I had my husband make excuses for why I couldn't take the call. I wanted no connection with anyone but my husband—it was a very isolating time. I needed direction from my own mom, but she had died many years ago. It was very difficult to not have my mother to care for me.

Although I couldn't eat much and had horrible anxiety, I knew I'd never hurt my babies. And I never felt suicidal. My mother had fought for her life against cancer and I knew I could never take my own. Before I had my babies, I put myself through college and graduate school and was the principal of a private school. I loved my work and took pride in the fact that I did so well for myself at a young age. I am social and like to be stimulated intellectually. Here I was, without my job. Who was I? What would become of me? All those years of hard work and now I was wrist-deep in poop. It was absolutely the right decision for our family for me to stay home, but it was also the hardest thing for me to adjust to. My family and friends felt helpless. Everyone was very worried about me, but one "friend" accused me of not loving my children. Supportive, wasn't she? I was convinced at the height of my PPD that my son hated me. But my wonderful pediatrician kept assuring me that the babies would have no recollection of my depression.

Even with all my misery, I knew I would bond with my babies and I figured my relations with them and my love for them would override how awful I felt . . . if not when I had PPD, then afterward. I just believed God would not have given me these two children if I could not bond with them and love them. Having said that, I am more concerned now with my relationship with them—I know they model their own behavior after mine and I want to be the best model for them.

I heard a message on the radio, looking for women with PPD to participate in a university hospital study. I was included in this and saw a doctor who prescribed medication. After two months I started to feel better. It saved my life. Pride is not

> When I panic, God teach me patience. When I fear, teach me faith. When I doubt myself, teach me confidence. When I despair, teach me hope. When I lose perspective, show me the way back to love, back to life, back to You.
> —Rabbi Naomi Levy

involved in healing from PPD. I thank God every day that medication exists and enabled me to live with joy, peace, and serenity. But don't get me wrong; medicine is not my panacea. Therapy, reading, writing, and a lot of soul-searching go hand-in-hand with the medication. I also put a notice in our synagogue bulletin, asking for in-home help. I am deeply grateful to these women (and of course to my extraordinary husband) for helping me reclaim the woman I am.

Now That I've Recovered

Just looking at the twins each morning with gratitude, not despair . . . could there be any greater accomplishment? I now can love myself through my mothering. There are no awards or career moves that top those accomplishments. If I can come through the other side of PPD, I can come through any challenge as a mom.

ISABELLE
28, EDUCATIONAL TOY REPRESENTATIVE/AT-HOME MOM
SOUTH AUSTRALIA, AUSTRALIA

Looking back, I wish the antenatal class that had just touched on PPD would have covered it in more depth. I think I would have recognized my symptoms much sooner. Also, a lot of people thought I shouldn't take antidepressants because they'd turn me into a "zombie" or make me worse. If I had not heard this, I would have gone on medication sooner.

My depression started at seven weeks postpartum when I developed severe insomnia and was lucky to manage one or two hours of sleep per night. Even when I had friends or family stay overnight to watch the twins so I could catch up on sleep, I could not. I became obsessed with sleep and thought if only I could sleep, everything would improve. But sleeping tablets wore off quickly and I'd be up all night. I became totally emotionally and physically drained. I had at least one serious bout of crying a day.

I looked at myself in the mirror and could barely recognize the image. I wondered if I would ever look happy again. I became fearful of going to bed because I knew I wasn't going to sleep. Then I dragged myself out of bed in the morning because I didn't want my day to start. I was exhausted when I'd hardly done a thing. I seemed to run on autopilot, managing to complete basic baby tasks because I had to. One morning I woke up and thought, "I don't want to be here anymore." I never contemplated suicide, but I was scared that if it got any worse, I might. I asked my husband to make sure I was never left alone.

I couldn't see that things would ever get better. It didn't matter what anyone told me, I couldn't think positively. People would try to do nice things to cheer me up, and it was all I could do just to smile and thank them. Laughing was practically impossible for me and even when my favorite songs were on the radio, I would not sing. I couldn't shake the deep down sadness.

I found a doctor through a local community health center. Although she doesn't specialize in PPD, she said she had patients with it all the time. I was prescribed antidepressants and sleeping medication. After just ten days, I started to feel better. During the nights I had plenty of rotating support from my mom, mother-in-law, husband, and a good friend. The multiple birth association also sent someone once a week. Thank goodness I read that article about PPD on the Internet! It described exactly how I was feeling. I realized I had a problem that just wasn't going to go away on its own and it encouraged me to seek help.

> So many people believe in you. Make sure you're one of them.
>
> —Unknown

The biggest thing that helped was just talking about it. The more I talked, the better I felt. Most people were more understanding than I thought they would be, as most had either experienced PPD to some degree or knew someone who had. I realized I wasn't alone. Many mothers were going through the same thing.

Now That I've Recovered

I am much more understanding of other people's problems. I am more able to see both sides of a situation and think it through. I am much more confident about speaking my own mind and not keeping things bottled up. I have taken a position doing in-home selling of educational toys. I never thought I'd have the confidence to do this—but I get more confident with each party. I enjoy it!

⁓⊙⁓ MARY JANE ⊙⁓
33, AT-HOME MOM
MARYLAND, USA

I was petrified at the thought of having a baby. Everyone was so excited I was having twins, but I was even more petrified. And yet, I also thought having a baby would somehow "complete" me. Instead, I felt nothing toward them. Just a numbness that was so scary.

I had tremendous anger inside me while I suffered from PPD. I was mad at my husband, my parents, and God—even my two helpless babies. At one time or another I came close to shaking them. I hit one of them too hard when I burped her. She screamed. I screamed, "I'm sorry!" over and over and cried for hours. New moms are supposed to fall in love with their babies, yet I woke up every morning praying that one of them would be dead. It is so hard to believe I could have ever felt these things. I'm such a different person now and my precious twins are in first grade, but I was suicidal for the first eight weeks postpartum. I wrote in my journal that the twins' would be better off with no mother than with me. PPD robbed me of joy during the twins' first eighteen months.

Eventually my doctor prescribed antidepressants. But when I stopped hiding my depression and talked to my sisters and a close friend, that's when I started to recover. They shared their stories of motherhood with me and even had some similar feelings. A huge burden was lifting off me. I should have taken the PPD discussions I heard while pregnant more seriously.

Now That I've Recovered

PPD is not just about being sad. There's a whole range of emotions you may feel. No matter how angry you might be, remember someone else felt that way, too. I am a much stronger person since recovering. Our family has a new two-year-old and these have been the happiest two years of my life. I could go on and on about how wonderful life is now . . . but I have three kids to take care of!

> A baby is God's opinion that the world should go on. Never will a time come when the most marvelous recent invention is as marvelous as a newborn baby.
>
> —Carl Sandburg

᠊᠊᠊ MONA ᠊᠊᠊
31, AT-HOME BINDERY BUSINESS OWNER
MINNESOTA, USA

My triplets were discharged on the same day. I had unrealistic expectations of new motherhood. I had no idea what to do or how to do it. I was overwhelmed and exhausted from not getting much sleep both before and after the babies arrived. I didn't feel like eating, showering, or taking care of the babies.

I felt like a baby-sitter. I did not feel any attachments and wondered about all these bonding moments most mothers and babies have from birth. I feared that I couldn't care for them or I might hurt them. I didn't know if I could be a mother. My husband couldn't understand my unhappiness and I couldn't explain it. I never sought professional help or medication. I went through PPD alone.

Although my husband couldn't understand how I felt, he was helpful and always there for me and for the babies. It just took time for me to learn how to take care of my babies. Slowly, we got into a routine, which helped.

Now That I've Recovered

I can now say I am proud of the mother that I have become. I love my children and love staying at home to raise them. My husband and I work hard to teach manners, respect, kindness, and gentleness. Our house is very ordered and we still strongly believe in schedule and routine.

I'm involved in a support group for mothers of multiples. With every hardship I have faced, I grow and become stronger. I also have a better understanding of what is important in life.

Take one day at a time and don't feel guilty or selfish for the feelings you have. They are your feelings—not right or wrong. Establishing routines helps eliminate stress. Remember, PPD is brought on by hormone changes and it won't last forever. In no way does it reflect on what kind of mother you can become.

~ MERYL ~
28, AT-HOME MOM
ILLINOIS, USA

My son had colic. If it wasn't hard enough to have two babies at once, we had to have one with colic. This was a complete nightmare. He cried from the moment he was awake until he went to sleep—for nine months! Everyone gave us suggestions, but there was nothing that helped. The doctor switched his formula so many times. I had no idea that my babies would take up every single minute of my life. I could not even shower or go to the bathroom. This was more work than I had to do at my job—at least I got to go home at night then, but this was 24/7, with no relief in sight.

I gave up my entire life for those babies. No time to go out anymore. So little sleep. No time for friends or even my husband. This was a huge adjustment. We were newlyweds, but we didn't have much time together alone. The first year of their life we only went out a few times by ourselves. My son's crying was so awful that my husband and I fought a lot about it. I was jealous that he got to go to work and I had to listen to my son wail all day. When my husband told me to get out of the house and take a break, I just wanted to sleep. He knew I was depressed.

Having had depression before, I thought I would get better with time. But I didn't. I knew I would get through this because it was up to me to take care of the kids. Even if I were miserable for the rest of my life, I would take care of them. I cried a lot and my husband said he'd never seen me so unhappy. I was so tired all the time, and had absolutely no sex drive, but I felt pressured by my husband to have sex.

I felt as if I were in a dark hole and couldn't get out. Hopelessness. The worst feeling I have ever experienced. I thought I was an awful person to deserve this. I called a local hospital to seek a psychiatrist. He prescribed an antidepressant and it helped me feel so much better. I had stayed cooped up in the house for days at a time. Getting fresh air every day helped. The best times were when the kids were finally in bed for the evening and my husband and I could spend time together—just watching TV or a movie. And I joined a group on the Internet for depression. I met a lot of wonderful people there and could vent my feelings if I needed to do that.

Now That I've Recovered

Raising my twins is a huge accomplishment. Getting through PPD was the hardest time of my life. I've learned so much and now I hope to help other mothers get through it. You don't have to feel like this. There is a solution.

Thoughts for a Better Day

I believe there should be some system in place to catch PPD early. Hospitals could set up home visits for every mom. OB/GYNs and pediatricians need to screen mothers for depression after a few weeks postpartum. And before delivery, OB/GYNs should rate each woman for her potential risk of developing PPD.

> List a minimum of five things to be grateful for each night. Become aware of all the wonderful people, modern conveniences, and simple pleasures you previously took for granted.

This illness also needs to be discussed in depth at birthing classes. Expectant moms need to set up support with other mothers of babies and young children before the baby is born—especially moms who've been in the work world a long time. They need that new network, because once depressed, it's hard to find or set up a network of peer support.

—Claire, 38, At-Home Mom
Maine, USA

CHAPTER 9

Mothers Looking for Their Maternal Instinct

After nine months of pregnancy most mothers expect to fall instantly in love when their new baby arrives. So it is understandable that the mothers in Chapter Nine were alarmed that instead of instant love, they felt detachment, indifference. Mothers felt guilty from these unexpected emotions and worried that they lacked "maternal instinct"—that they were somehow flawed. They identified these feelings as a factor of falling into postpartum depression.

The good news is that once they recovered they would ultimately bond with their babies and indeed experience the intensely emotional connection, the special mother and child union of a blossoming family.

✦ TOULA ✦
32, CORPORATE EXECUTIVE
MISSOURI, USA

After my mother-in-law left from staying with us for a week and a half after delivery, I was frightened. I could never nap when the baby napped. I became overwhelmed with the fear of being responsible for his life. I had never imagined how hard motherhood would be. I really didn't think I'd ever be a mother. I didn't have maternal instincts or the desire, really. I thought, what the heck am I doing? I know nothing about babies. Had zero experience.

I had feelings of helplessness; especially not being able to get things done, such as balance the checkbook, cook meals, or clean house. The baby was too demanding. I also felt I lost my sex appeal, that now I was just a mom, not a woman desired by my husband. My role had changed.

I thought about going to a therapist, but I never did seek professional help. I don't know many people who have gone to therapy. I began to recover from PPD when I started regularly exercising and getting out to see friends. Finally, getting a routine down also helped. When I was really stressed, I'd take long baths. And deep breathing yoga exercises helped. Spending time alone with my husband became a must—even if it was just to cuddle or have a glass of wine together.

Now That I've Recovered

I try not to look back at my old life. Life has changed—and there are new challenges ahead. My new life has more meaning and importance now that I'm a parent.

CRYSTAL

30, AUDIOLOGIST
PENNSYLVANIA, USA

I consider myself very upbeat and I have an extremely good sense of humor. So I knew something was very wrong, even before I left the hospital. I was glad to finally meet my little guy, especially since I swore he was a boy right from the beginning. I knew from the get-go that this was not the "baby blues" that relatives assured me it was. I was making a 180-degree turn from my normal personality.

I cried all day, didn't want my husband to leave my side, needed to have someone always near me, and thought I'd made a huge mistake becoming a mother. I had illogical thoughts. I thought I was not the maternal woman that I had assumed I was.

My insurance company referred a psychiatrist, who thankfully saw me immediately. We discussed medication and she asked if I would be opposed to it. I told her she could hook me up to an IV if that would make the feelings go away. She also sent me to a social worker for counseling. She stressed that I had to remember it would get better, that I must repeat those words a thousand times.

Luckily in my case, the medication kicked in very quickly. Within a week and a half I began not to dread every sunrise and began to see the proverbial "light at the end of the tunnel." After just three weeks on medication, the social worker told me I was the complete opposite of the person she had met only a month before.

Thoughts for a Better Day

Watching my son grow is the best thing I have ever experienced in my life, even with the PPD. When my son looks at me, and smiles because he thinks I am the greatest thing in the world, it melts my heart. Women need to know that even with PPD, you'll feel like that, too.

I discuss PPD with anyone who will listen. I can name at least two friends who likely had PPD and never sought help until it almost destroyed their marriages. I am not embarrassed because I had depression, nor for the fact that I was put on an antidepressant.

It's amazing the number of people who have told me, "I can't believe you were depressed. You're always laughing and smiling." But depression can affect anyone. Our society needs to change how it views PPD and all depressions. If everyone realized how many people they knew had seen a mental health professional or were on antidepressants, they would be amazed!

⤚◠ BRACHA ◠⤙
30, DOULA
CALIFORNIA, USA

When my baby was born, I secretly wondered if I were worthy of motherhood. I kept waiting for that "wonderful mothering instinct" to kick in. I experienced "nonbonding" when she was born. Having a demanding, colicky baby was a shocker. I had such an enjoyable pregnancy, and all I heard was how wonderful it was all going to be. It took me many weeks to get used to my daughter's demands, but eventually it did get better. I've always been highly irritable and emotional my whole life, so of course any physical hormonal changes caused me to become excitable (periods, pregnancy, postpartum . . . gee, I can't wait for menopause!).

The dreams I had of harming my baby were the scariest, and they're what caused me not to admit to anyone that I didn't have motherly feelings. Yet, through it all, I never neglected or ignored my baby. I was protective of her. When she was a couple of months old and started to react to the world and smile, that's when I really started to love her and look forward to being with her every day. I did not seek any professional help or take medication.

I have kept a diary since I was twelve. Being able to write down my true feelings without being judged has always been cathartic for me. My husband and I also rent movies whenever we have the time and money to sit back and enjoy a few hours of distraction from reality. It helped us to have that to look forward to and we still do it today.

Now That I've Recovered

Since having my second (and last) child, I have discovered the fascinating and rewarding world of being a labor and support doula. I have helped many other women going through PPD. I think all women need to know they are not alone in their doubts, and I regularly share my new mother memories with moms I support. I think it helps them get through those rough first weeks.

All you can do as a new mom is realize that eventually the babies do get older and it's amazing to watch them be excited by their growing world perception. Find other moms you can relate to and find professional help if new parenthood is too much to deal with. Remember . . . this, too, shall pass, and our children do look up to us as they grow. I'm very proud of my children!

GLENDA
34, AT-HOME MOM
NEW YORK, USA

My baby boy was only one month old and I felt I had made the wrong decision to have a child. I didn't want to take care of him anymore. I felt ashamed, fatigued, overwhelmed, depressed, lonely, and angry. I lost interest in all things I used to enjoy. I didn't sleep more than two hours in a few weeks. I cried for no reason and had anxiety attacks. I lost weight quickly.

Everyone wanted me to pull myself together and "snap out of it," but I knew there was more to this. This was not me. I planned for this child and looked forward to his birth with open arms . . . so how could I be feeling these horrible things? One day as my husband was going to work when the baby was two months old, I considered putting him up for adoption. I was an unfit mother and was dragging my family down. This "decision" made me even more depressed.

I looked at my infant son—he was so beautiful and he just wanted me to love him and hold him. In my heart I wanted that, too, but something was so wrong. I felt empty of any emotions. Relatives helped me until my husband came home from work. I had no desire to hold my baby, but I would; and gather up any emotions of love I could to let my baby know that I knew he wasn't the problem. Something else was wrong with me.

One day I had convulsions and collapsed. I had stopped sleeping and eating and my body just shut down. The medication my doctor prescribed would take about a month to start working, and I continued taking it for eight months. I also received tremendous support from a local postpartum resource center.

> I wrote notes to myself and taped them all over the house. Examples were: "I am a wonderful and nurturing mother," "I am a great wife," "My husband loves me so much," "I have terrific children," and so on. These little notes helped quite a bit. Especially in triggering positive "self-talk."
>
> —Molly, 35, At-Home Mom
> Virginia, USA

Thoughts for a Better Day

Well, the happy ending is I got better. I am so in love with my son, who is now two years old. My marriage is healthier and happier. I now volunteer to help mothers who are suffering from PPD. This affliction is a valid illness that is one hundred percent curable. Remember . . . you are not alone, and you are not to blame. Find someone you can really trust with your craziest thoughts. All this insanity is only temporary. Mothers with PPD are faced with the stigma of mental health issues, and their dim belief in their ability to overcome this painful condition. You are not losing your mind. Take small steps, one day at a time, and you will get well.

PARIS

29, SPEECH PATHOLOGIST
NEBRASKA, USA

I had never had any depression before—not even any PMS mood swings. I'm usually a very optimistic and easygoing person. So I was surprised to encounter this. I thought motherhood would make me feel instantly fulfilled. Instead, I felt exhausted and detached from any aspect of normal that I felt before the baby. I worried that I didn't feel an instant and fulfilling love for my son. I would lie in bed between feedings, thinking, "I should go check to see if he's breathing." But then I would think if he didn't make it, it wasn't meant to be. Now I can't believe I felt this way. I check him more at night (he's two) now than I did when he was a newborn.

I was very emotional and had terrible mood swings. I couldn't remember which breast I breast-fed with from hour to hour. My husband made a chart and kept track for me. One time I cried for two hours because I couldn't decide whether to use one product or another on my son's diaper rash. Another time we were shopping and when my husband went to the car to get the coupons I suddenly realized I was alone with the baby. I just started bawling. It took fifteen minutes for my husband to calm me down in the store.

Overall, I felt as if I were in a hole of sleeplessness that I would never climb out of, but when I talked to family or friends, I would always say how great everything was going. I kept my feelings a secret. Time fostered my recovery. I learned to accept the difficulties of being a new mother. Eventually, as my son became less demanding, I had time to rest and catch up on sleep. My husband was the biggest support. He stayed calm and tried to help in every aspect. He never made me feel stupid or ashamed, but instead he rolled with the punches and took care of the house, the baby, and me.

Now That I've Recovered

Our family is very close and my son is well-adjusted and full of energy. I just had another baby boy and had a couple of days of baby blues, but no depression. I experienced joy and euphoria with this baby that I never experienced with my first son. This time around I had plenty of help lined up so I would not become overwhelmed.

Join the local chapter of M.O.M.S. (Moms Offering Moms Support). Finding a support group helps tremendously. There is probably a local chapter near you, or see their website, momsclub.org.

If you are experiencing PPD, don't keep it secret. Find a support group. It helps so much to know you are not alone—other mothers really are feeling the same way.

─∽⊙∾ TESSA ∽⊙∾─
30, SOCIAL WORKER
ONTARIO, CANADA

I felt terribly concerned about my relationship with my daughter. I went through the motions—fed her and bathed her—but I had to force myself. I really just wanted to curl up in a corner. My husband ended up getting up with her at night once I started medication and sleeping pills. I felt so guilty. I kept apologizing to my daughter that she didn't have a better mom. The anxiety was the worst part of my PPD. I didn't relax for a minute. I had severe insomnia. As soon as I shut my eyes, my thoughts would start racing.

I read many books about newborns and I was sure she had every illness in them. Everyone told me to trust my instincts, but I didn't have any. I read a lot of conflicting information. It sent my head spinning and I couldn't make decisions. I couldn't get food down and didn't cook. Thank God for my mother-in-law, who cooked for us. I didn't feel happy or sad. I didn't feel love or hate. Just nothing. It was the worst "nonfeeling" I've ever had in my life. Rarely leaving the house made me think of it as a prison. I never had any hurtful thoughts toward my baby, but I worried I'd go into some sort of catatonic state.

My husband took two months off work to help me, and my mother-in-law was with us constantly. My own mother accused me of using PPD as a crutch. It was horrible. From then on my husband and mother-in-law were the only ones I relied on. My mother-in-law even cut her vacation time short because of me. I truly feel I wouldn't have made it through the experience without her. I wanted to pack my things and disappear because everyone would have been better off without me, but I wanted to be a part of my daughter's life. I truly wanted to get better for her and return to the person I once was.

I went to a PPD support group, where I discovered I had the worst case of the group—that made me feel even worse at first. But I got brave and went back several weeks later and met a woman whose experience was similar to mine. She was in the recovery phase and doing quite well. She helped me more than she'll ever know.

Now That I've Recovered

The fact that I've survived PPD and am now a happy stay-at-home mom is my biggest accomplishment. My daughter is now two and a half and I'm pregnant again. I'm scared, but I know that if PPD arises again it's only temporary and I'll get through it. My advice is to seek help with the first sign that something is "wrong." If you do have PPD, know that with a strong desire to get better, with support, and if necessary, with the help of medication, you can recover.

ZOEY
38, SCIENTIFIC COORDINATOR
CALIFORNIA, USA

I was obsessed with the relationship I had with my daughter. I was so scared we would never bond. When I held her, she would stiffen and arch her back. I was so sure that meant she couldn't stand to have me hold her. I worried people would scrutinize me; they could tell my daughter was miserable with me. Mothers would say my baby could sense how tense I was and it was making it hard for her. God, how I resented that.

The only thing that helped her was to nurse. I used to feel so apologetic and weak that I couldn't do anything else for her. When angry, I would handle her roughly and feel so terrible about it. I knew I was a terrible mother. Three weeks postpartum, I joined a PPD support group. The leader said it didn't matter if I couldn't control my baby's crying. She said it didn't matter!

I began therapy with a social worker as well, and she actually said I was doing a good job and was a good mother. I had no idea because I was so deep into my negative view of myself. I did not take any medication. The PPD support group helped me and I reached out a lot. My family was frustrated and annoyed that I didn't "snap out of it." My friends never understood the full magnitude of my depression. I found a day care provider and returned to work. Just being back to where I felt adequate helped lift my depression immensely.

Now That I've Recovered

I have a lot of peace and confidence. I'm a wonderful mother and I've become more spiritual. My kids are my inspiration.

ᴼᴼ SONYA ᴼᴼ
34, DOULA
NEW YORK, USA

Everyone prepares for labor in childbirth class, but there's not much out there for the transition to motherhood. I never thought about colic or a baby that did not sleep. With my son born in June, I thought we would take walks, sit outside, and relax. Quite the opposite was true.

I could barely shower, make a bed, eat, or go to the bathroom. I thought I'd accomplish so much on maternity leave, but I felt so useless. I didn't love my baby. What was wrong with me? Here I had been trying to conceive for three years, wanting this baby, yet I loved my dog much more. I felt I was the worst mother. Then I'd have guilty feelings. I wanted my life back.

If one more person told me how cute my baby was or said, "Don't you love him?" I would die inside. How do you tell anyone that you despise this baby?

Although I thought I wasn't a good mother, I knew I would take care of him and never hurt him. But I hated being a mom. I did scream and swear at him once and I understood how some of "those" mothers threw their babies out windows, or shook and hurt them. It made sense now. Those poor women.

I never sought help, as I didn't know I was ill and I just thought I was a bad mother. I guess you could say my mom was my biggest therapist. We were very close and she never judged me, just stood by me and followed up every day. She made meals and stopped by to give me a break. My grandparents would stop by, too, and say what a great mom I was. (Come to think of it, they still do—five years later!)

I don't remember a turning point. Just one day I had a good day and felt better. I became more confident as a mother and felt I actually loved my son. Each day I woke up I questioned my abilities, so when we had good days it was confidence-building.

Now That I've Recovered

That was the most trying situation in my life. I came through and I'm proud of myself, but I should have asked for help. I have since become a doula. Now I help other women. I never thought I'd survive, let alone support others. Now when I walk into their homes and they cry, I tell them my story and it helps them. They know they are not alone and they are relieved.

Thoughts for a Better Day

If you are suffering from PPD, remember the process to recovery seems to be two steps forward and one step back. The bad days don't mean that you've lost all your hard-won progress. When those days come, accept them as inevitable and recognize them as survivable. Focus on the progress you are making.

—Violet, 30, At-Home Mom
California, USA

CHAPTER 10

Mothers with High Expectations

Almost all of the mothers in this book had high expectations of motherhood. We all expected this to be the happiest time of our life. The buildup of anticipation to the expected period of bliss after a baby arrives seems universal. All the images we've seen in the media while growing up—scenes of mothers holding their calm babies so serene and fulfilled, scenes of a clean home with dinner on the table as Mommy and baby wait for Daddy to come home from work—feed our expectations. The mother in our fantasies is always well rested. (After all, isn't new motherhood like vacation? You get maternity leave!) How hard could taking care of a tiny infant be?

On top of these fantasies and expectations many of the women in Chapter Ten strived to be "perfect." Every element of our life has to be perfect and in control. It all leads up to a very crude "reality check" as we shockingly discover how new motherhood is very much an out-of-control experience. A new infant is incredibly demanding 24/7. We experienced the overwhelming changes and adjustments of what new motherhood is really like. Unexpectedly, we became clinically depressed at the one time of our life when we expected to be the opposite—to be blissfully happy.

We all survived the fast, steep drops and sharp turns of this scary roller-coaster ride . . . and in the end, we all gained much wisdom from the lessons learned on the tracks.

~⊙ CARMEN ⊙~
31, ADMINISTRATIVE ASSISTANT
MANITOBA, CANADA

I prided myself on being an organized, self-sufficient person. After my daughter was born, I realized my life had changed in ways I did not conceive possible. The schedule I thought I'd adhere to meant nothing. This is hard to take for a type A personality. It was hard to "let go" and accept things. I intended to use cloth diapers. That ended fairly quickly. I vowed never to let our daughter sleep in our bed. That changed. Without realizing it, I was going to be Super Mom. I wasn't and I never will be. I didn't share my feelings with family or friends. I was irritable and emotional. Thank God I never took it out on my daughter—that never entered my mind. My husband took the brunt of the emotional roller coaster I was on.

I felt overwhelmed and had suicidal thoughts—but really I just wanted to be replaced by a mother who was more competent. I wished I hadn't entered into this unknown, then I felt tremendous guilt over these thoughts. I dressed like a slob. I didn't bother with my hair or makeup. I felt lost in my own world.

I read an article about postpartum depression in *Self* magazine. After reading it, I was laughing and crying at the same time. The realization of what was wrong did wonders for me. I began to read as much as I could about it. I was not alone, and I was not crazy.

I relied on my husband and friends to help me recover. A few months after my baby was born, my friends insisted on taking me out for drinks for the evening. This was a huge step for me, and it did a world of good. Eventually, I started going to the mall with my daughter. Lots of moms hung out there.

Now That I've Recovered

I am back to work full-time, but I wish it were part-time. My relationship with my husband is back on track. If you have postpartum depression, try to adopt a "one day at a time" attitude. If you have clean underwear and your baby has clean clothes, you are doing great. If anyone wants to come over and visit, tell them to bring supper! Above all, don't be afraid to talk about it.

~~·⌒· Mercedes ·⌒·~~
35, Advertising Agency Creative Director
New South Wales, Australia

My expectations of motherhood were set by television commercials. All white softness and gurgles. Even though I heard that you'll never feel as tired as when you're a new mother, I believed I would be different. I was in charge of my destiny and no little baby could get the better of me. Wrong! I was never, not even once, able to nap when the baby slept. At night he slept at one or two hourly intervals for about seven months. I was never a good sleeper, but to be deprived of even the smallest amount is sheer torture.

I remember a friend's mother saying she would just kiss every inch of her babies over and over because she just adored them. I had no feelings for my baby. I had nowhere to run and no one who would understand. There was no way out. My escape was the Internet. I would stay up all night talking in chat rooms, reinventing myself. I felt entirely irrational. I call it my mad phase. I did things I don't remember. My doctor asked me if I was suicidal and I laughed and said absolutely not. But in the back of my mind, I believed the only way to end this overwhelming grayness would be to do it. Knowing the only option was to endure the depression or commit suicide just made the whole situation worse.

I gave up outside work and threw myself into my role as mother far more actively. Even though I didn't realize it, soon this role of motherhood was growing on me. I realized that almost everything I longed for was within my reach, but I was choosing other paths. I began doing arts and crafts with my son, and I finally started to bond with him. I gave up the Internet, and made myself interact with people face-to-face to restore my confidence socially.

> Every morning wake up and say, "Today I am going to be happy." At first you may not be feeling it, but one day your brain will get used to the idea. You'd be surprised how far the right thoughts will move you into a brighter reality.

Now That I've Recovered

Our family life is extremely happy now and I am fulfilled as a full-time mother. I proudly spread the word about postpartum depression to let all mothers from all walks of life know that they are indeed at risk.

~♥~ HOLLY ~♥~
36, RESEARCH OFFICER
SOUTH AUSTRALIA, AUSTRALIA

I have always been a perfectionist, a high achiever, one who needs a seal of approval from others and a need to feel in control. I can see now that this all clashes with having kids. I think my depression was caused partly by my desire to continue work, but this clashed with the feeling that a "good mother" should stay home with her kids. I know now that I'm definitely not a baby person—or maybe it's just because I had such a negative experience. It was hard to be on maternity leave with this little baby that is entirely your responsibility, but that you can't control.

My experience of the first year of motherhood was all unexpected. No one ever told us about any of it—how you might really feel—except for one couple. They looked like zombies most of the time after their first, and we assumed it was because they were the minority who couldn't cope. We now know they were trying to give us a realistic picture. Now when we try to do the same for others, people don't listen. It's like you're not supposed to shatter the frilly, gooey, fuzzy images of new motherhood with the reality of sleep deprivation, exhaustion, and frustration.

Looking back, I now notice that even on occasional days when I'd had a bad night's sleep and had been up with the kids two or three times I was quite irritable the next day. No wonder after one year of sleep deprivation I felt depressed. I sobbed my heart out. I mourned being far away from friends and family back in England. I felt humiliation and shame being rolled into a strange hospital on a stretcher after my baby came quickly at home. And I mourned the loss of my close relationship with my husband. I think the stress from frustration with the baby created anger between us. I was so exhausted I couldn't think straight. I'd do anything for my first born—total sacrifice. But with our second baby, I'd get frustrated and often felt like throwing her at the wall. I've never had as much patience with her, which of course caused great guilt.

On several occasions I asked for help, but it was never forthcoming. A child health nurse asked me—when I broke down at the clinic—if I had postnatal depression. But I didn't know yet what that was so I couldn't say yes or no. It ended there. I also was referred, by a PPD support group of past sufferers, to a psychiatric day clinic, but by then I had no confidence to go out anywhere in public with two kids. I finally found help through a Lifeline telephone helpline for confidential and anonymous help. This was the best help! For me it was nonjudgmental and available when it fit my schedule. I also saw a psychologist at work, but I'm not one for taking drugs so I never took any medication.

Now That I've Recovered

Lord, help me to remember that nothing is going to happen to me today that you and I together cannot handle.

—Unknown Author

I have really benefited from all the reading I've done about PPD. I now understand myself a lot better. It's been a journey deep into my personality. I now nurture my relationship with my husband and I want my kids to know it's okay not to be perfect. It is important to have fun. I know not to neglect my own needs. If I practice being a happy mother and we are happy parents, everything else will fall into place. A lot of women put themselves last and kids first to a fault. In the end it takes its toll. Be sure to take care of yourself.

Thoughts for a Better Day

One of the most frustrating things during this time was the mother image that is expected of all new mothers. If this book helps dispel the mother myth (the perfect fairy-tale mother) that alone is a step in the right direction! I think there is a small population of women who can transform their lives in a day. Becoming a mother has been a gradual process for me. Two years later, I can honestly say I'm a great mother. Maybe even better than some of those moms I was once envisioning . . . you know, the ones that look like they were born for motherhood. But for some of us, it takes time, adjustment, and support. It's a learning process, and your heart grows larger as your children grow and you get to know who they are. I would not trade motherhood for the world. I am trying for a second, but if PPD happens again, I'll be prepared this time.

—Iris, 35, Portfolio Manager
Massachusetts, USA

SHEENA
38, WRITER
CALIFORNIA, USA

My expectations of motherhood were ridiculous. I had absolutely no idea how stressful it was to maintain the constant vigilance newborns demand. On the other hand, I don't think anyone can really appreciate or anticipate all this without being a parent. It's something you really have to experience for yourself. I felt very committed to my daughter. I knew I absolutely had to protect her, but the real love and pleasure in her company came later.

I sensed the depression coming on around day three, the night before I left the hospital. Just a couple of days later I felt so overwhelmed and disoriented that I actually asked my husband if we could give our daughter to a couple from our infertility support group who were looking for a child to adopt. This was one of the worst moments of my life. I thought I must be a bad mother who didn't love her child.

The depression peaked when she was about a month old. I was filled with anxiety by the sense that I had so much to learn and by feelings of grief because my life changed so irrevocably. I was terrified that I'd never recover my old self, that I'd never feel relaxed or happy again. I could usually fall asleep after nursing her in the middle of the night. Mornings, I'd wake up fairly optimistic, but by two P.M. I was ready to die of grief and the feeling of entrapment. I had a panic attack in a store while holding my baby in my arms. This scared me to death. In the middle of a department store I had to talk myself back to reality. I began to have mild fantasies about tossing my baby down in the backyard. I felt so stupid. Here I had struggled so hard to have a baby, and now that I had her, I didn't want her.

I never did seek professional help, but I did join a mother's group that was very helpful because by then I was already improving. When my daughter turned five weeks old, she looked in my eyes and smiled for the first time. I smiled back. She smiled back again; maintaining eye contact, and I started crying. For the first time I felt like we made conscious contact with each other. It just made a huge difference to me and I began to recover.

Now That I've Recovered

Eventually my marriage deteriorated, but I am much stronger and smarter for the experience. I left my dead-end job and now enjoy my writing career, and volunteering at my daughter's school library. I recommend that new mothers hire a doula to come over every day the first two weeks after childbirth, and a few times a week for the next month. This makes a great shower gift. Also, instead of cute little outfits, ask friends and family to bring dinner once a week for a month. You're working 24/7 nourishing someone, and you need to be nourished yourself. Accept help. Postpartum hormonal changes do weird things to everyone. Your baby will settle down eventually, and you'll feel more like yourself again.

~⊙ WINONA ⊙~

27, AT-HOME MOM
TEXAS, USA

My expectations of new motherhood were nowhere near reality. Nobody ever told me how much work a newborn would be. I was frustrated that my husband didn't help more at night, even though he couldn't do much since I was breast-feeding. I felt this intense need to know every detail of the baby's care (burps, diaper changes, sleep position), but at the same time I felt like escaping and sleeping for days. My mother and mother-in-law both seemed clueless as to how to support me. Neither seemed to relate to my anxiety or loneliness.

When my daughter cried and I was unable to console her, I doubted if she loved me, and I'd wonder if I'd made a mistake by having a baby. One mistake for sure was reading a book that emphasized establishing a routine with your newborn. I had unrealistic expectations that led to a lot of anxiety and frustrations. As my anxiety grew, I felt depression creeping in. I started to feel helpless and out of control, acting very emotional and sensitive, especially to the outside world. I remember watching television and feeling disgusted at all the violence, sex, and lack of morals. I felt an intense need to protect my baby from the world.

I cried every day for eight weeks. My husband would ask me what was wrong, but I couldn't come up with an answer. It felt purely hormonal. The more exhausted I became, the more my mind raced. The level of anxiety was higher than I'd ever felt before. I considered seeing a therapist, but decided to wait and see if the depression lifted.

I have two wonderful friends who had experienced PPD and they were so encouraging and loving. They would remind me of how important my job as a mother was, and would give me understanding and reassurances that my depression wouldn't last forever. I also tried to make it to our women's Bible study once a week.

Coming out of depression was a gradual process. I began to make an effort to get out of the house every Saturday and leave the baby with my husband, who would bottle-feed her my expressed milk. I'd take a drive, long walk, or long bubble bath—alone. Once I had made "me time" on a daily basis, the depression began to subside.

Now That I've Recovered

My initial sense of being overwhelmed has faded, and I am no longer extremely anxious taking care of my baby. I have increased confidence in myself as a mother, and have peace that God will give me wisdom as a parent. My depression has taken me to a deeper level of faith and trust in God, and has made me a stronger person.

Thoughts for a Better Day

> I can do all things through Christ who strengthens me.
>
> —Philippians 4:13

I would not wish PPD on my worst enemy. I've been to hell and back, but now I'm a stronger, more insightful person. Do not suffer alone. You are not going crazy . . . you'll get better. You are the best mother your baby can have and you are doing an excellent job!

—Clara, 28, Administrative Officer
South Australia, Australia

CHAPTER 11

Mothers Adjusting After
Fast-Paced Careers

Prior to giving birth, I was—like many of the women in Chapter Eleven—in a fast-paced, pressure-filled career . . . an environment where I thrived. I enjoyed the camaraderie of my coworkers and the sense of daily accomplishment derived from helping clients through their advertising campaigns. Most of all, I was very, very busy and the days flew by.

But I, like many mothers who will get postpartum depression, experienced a sudden, drastic change of pace as a new mother. We no longer visited with coworkers and clients. Instead we were in an empty house, surrounded by four walls. The isolation became unbearable. Transitioning from closing deals to changing diapers and from rooms full of people to one tiny baby was difficult. Time shifted right down to slow gear. In fact, with the lack of structure in the day, time seemed to stand still.

The identity crisis began . . . am I career woman or a mother? Can I be both? Should I be both? Part of the recovery process occurs as we make decisions about how to balance our roles.

⁓꧁ Marianne ꧂⁓
36, At-Home Mom
Ontario, Canada

I know I did not want to return to work after my baby was born. I believed it was important for a parent to be home during the all-important early years. However, the realization that I was not going back to a career that I had established over eleven years was jarring. My job was predictable. My baby was not! Babies' schedules don't fit a day-timer, and I was not prepared for the responsibility and the role of mom.

I was the good girl child: straight-A student, graduated summa cum laude, won a scholarship, graduated with a B.A. in English literature with high distinction, never did drugs, and always met my expectations—or maybe I should say my parents' expectations. No one, certainly not my mother, would ever think I could get postpartum depression. Maybe this explains why she burst into my room after one particular crying spell and screamed at me to "snap out of it." To this day, I remember thinking she was right . . . whatever made me think I could raise a child? I questioned my very existence and worthiness. My mother always belittled my depression.

I was the first one of my group of friends to have a child, so no one could relate to my feelings of depression and helplessness. Sleep—what was that? Every baby noise propelled me out of bed and left me hovering around her bassinet. I was nervous and weepy. A total insomniac. I couldn't sleep—what if anything happened to her? I'd never forgive myself. I was afraid to sleep in case she needed me. Afraid to shower in case she cried. Afraid to do any task for fear I'd leave it undone. I would call my husband at his office, hysterical, and he'd feel helpless. I lost interest in sex. I lost interest in everything. My husband asked me if there wasn't somebody out there I could talk to about this.

Through a helpline for moms, I connected with a new mother support group. Through meeting and befriending these six mothers— all with, to some extent, similar problems—I was transformed. It gave me something to look forward to every week.

Let go. Let God.

Now That I've Recovered

I try to look at things with humor—find the innate absurdities and laugh. I'm now more aware of the need to laugh at life, to look at things more positively.

ERIN
41, MUSICIAN
NEW MEXICO, USA

After my daughter was born, I was overwhelmed by feelings as though I had lost my identity. I had a sense that my baby daughter owned every cell of my body. The most difficult part of her early infancy was the feeling that time lost any rhythm. Suddenly there was no day or night. The baby consumed every moment and interrupted every thought. I sat for hours and hours nursing her, hoping for the chance to complete a one-armed meal such as tuna eaten from its can with a spoon. I felt like a confined cat. My lifeline to sanity existed in the form of a cordless phone. I couldn't wait for my husband to come home at night. I felt exhausted and desperate to have time alone. There was, of course, sweet times those early weeks, but the bulk of it was very difficult. Isolation is typical for postpartum women who don't live near families. What I needed was a community of women to support me—just like in giving birth. I was birthing my new self, and I needed guides, helpers, angels.

I was filled with thoughts of me as the villain, hurting my baby. I cannot emphasize enough how painful these thoughts were and how I also knew that I was absolutely not capable of hurting my baby. I adored my little girl. I now understand the pain of mental illness. I feel so much compassion for those who suffer. After all, if you have a broken leg, no big deal. But if you have a broken mind . . .

> Every time a scary thought rears its ugly head, take a long, deep breath, focus on the breath and this thought, "I am not my thoughts. I am not my thoughts." This will stop provoking fear in you. Gradually the bad thoughts will fade away like the refrain of a song.

I went back to work at the store and cradled my baby snuggly to me. We were no longer alone all day with my terrifying thoughts because I talked to people in the store. I felt a huge burden lift from me. I began to heal.

BIANCA
27, AT-HOME MOM
TEXAS, USA

I was a full-time graduate student with two jobs before I became a mother and homemaker. Coming from an academic lifestyle, I was used to living by deadlines and schedules. A life without due dates and structure seemed like too much for me. I didn't know how to begin doing anything when nothing had to be done.

My expectations of the demands of a new baby were fairly realistic, but I didn't realize how time-consuming it would be. I thought I'd be able to catch up on my scrapbooking and other projects. My husband expected me to always get up with the baby at night, plus keep our home spotless. I was too tired to do it, lethargic from becoming a light sleeper, and I just wanted to sit on the couch all day. I used to enjoy playing the piano—now this and other favorite activities held no interest for me.

Sometimes I felt resentful that the baby changed my life. I didn't fall in love with him like I thought I would, and I wondered why. My depression lasted from one month to four months postpartum, and I didn't tell anyone about it. I withdrew from my husband and being new to town, I had no friends nearby. The thought of spending all day, every day with my new baby made me feel hopeless. I could see years stretching out in front of me with nothing to look forward to but the next feeding. I wished I could go to sleep and not wake up. Just stop existing.

When we purchased a car for me, I realized I wasn't so trapped. I could see the possibility of life with my baby. We started to go to the local gym, and I made myself work out . . . it helped tremendously. I started keeping a calendar and looking for things to put on it. At first it was little things like "do laundry" on Thursdays or "go shopping before baby's nap." The little things helped me feel more in control. Then I aimed for things further out that I could look forward to, like my parents' Christmas visit. At first I focused on each day, because the "future" was too much for me. But eventually, I could expand my view and look up and out at life again.

Now That I've Recovered

I now have an active, cheerful three-year-old. We had another baby with no depression afterward. I'm back in control of my life and own my own business. I appreciate my husband more and know he'll give me support if I just ask.

Don't hide and deal with

Make "done" lists instead of "to do" lists. Write down each accomplishment, such as: fed baby, showered, did laundry, read baby a book, etc. . . . These lists will give you a sense of success and accomplishment. Your self-confidence will return. It just takes time.

PPD alone. Talk to someone—your husband, your doctor, or a friend. Let them help you! You deserve to be happy and to feel good about your life and yourself.

⇜ Natasha ⇝
32, At-Home Mom
New York, USA

Now That I've Recovered

I recovered and had a second child, and I have a new philosophy: Life gives us lessons to learn. We continue to have those lessons until we learn from them. Afterward another lesson appears. It is a never-ending cycle that makes us live more fully. Now, each time life throws me a curve, I throw it right back. I charge ahead and deal with any situation because I believe there is something in each of the lessons from which I can learn and grow.

Thoughts for a Better Day

I have always been raised to be independent and ambitious. I was taught to depend on myself for happiness, and not a man, and definitely, not to start a family until I was ready. Now I've had a baby, and according to the cultural norm I should be completely happy staying home and taking care of my baby. That should be my sole fulfillment. Can you see the catch here? The idea of staying home and having my life revolve around someone else goes against every expectation for myself I had been raised with. Remembering this has helped me conquer the guilt over not being "happy" as a stay-at-home mom.

—Eydie, 32, Dean of Student Services
California, USA

CHAPTER 12

Mothers Overcoming Anger Toward Their Husbands

Time after time, the mothers in this book have expressed the gratitude they felt as their husbands cared for them through this burdensome illness. To those husbands who had faith that their wives would one day get better and were there to support them through all their anxieties, worries, and torrents of tears, we salute you. Strong, faithful, understanding husbands were crucial to mothers recovering from postpartum depression.

The women in Chapter Twelve were not so lucky. Without feeling that dependable support they so desperately needed, they lashed out in anger and frustration at their spouses. These women had husbands who—far from being supportive—wanted their wives to continue keeping the house clean, having food on the table, and having sex. They would not accept that their wives were suffering from a disabling mental illness.

Postpartum depression will test a couple's marriage. But once the storm has passed, the couple's relationship is hopefully stronger and more able to withstand whatever the future brings.

ᵔᵒᏺ Monique ᏺᵒᵔ

32, Customer Service Representative
Ohio, USA

I felt so overwhelmed and out of control. Like I was a volcano about to erupt. With no help from my husband who works a lot, I felt all alone and miserable.

I also worried about my ability to take care of my baby. She was colicky, and it seemed that I had depression even worse because of it. I felt like a terrible mother because I had visions of throwing her out the window or balcony, just to make the crying go away.

I felt resentment toward my husband and withdrew from him. When I finally would get some free time to myself, I didn't want to be touched, but he would want sex. By the time he came home from work, I'd just want to pass out from exhaustion.

A marriage therapist diagnosed me as depressed, but did not specifically indicate PPD. My physician prescribed antidepressants. They took two to three weeks to start helping me. I primarily relied on my email friendships for support.

Now That I've Recovered

I now offer support and advice to moms-to-be. I let them know I am here to help them if they need me. This helps me heal, knowing that I can help others through my own experience.

You are not alone. Join a mothers' support group. Ask for help. I wish I had done so earlier, but I've learned through my own experience that you can't be a new mom and do it all. Unless you don't care about your sanity!

⤙ Ursula ⤚
34, Registered Nurse
England, U.K.

With this baby I seemed to have a lot more anger in addition to the melancholy, and I directed it toward my husband. I would shout and scream at him and then, about four months into this illness, I lost all my fight and became very withdrawn, spending a large portion of the day crying.

At my angriest, I put my hand through a glass door panel and cut my palm and wrist. I had especially hard times at night. Finally, I was referred to a crisis response for after-hours care. It was reassuring to know my husband or I could call someone who would visit us or provide us with phone contact. I also saw a psychiatrist for eighteen months and an antidepressant was prescribed. I used music to calm me, especially when I could feel myself getting uptight with my husband. If I felt aggression brewing toward him, I used relaxation techniques, including slow, deep breathing and imagining myself somewhere else. It didn't always work, but he also learned when things were getting bad and removed himself from the situation.

Going back to work provided my greatest support and healing.

Now That I've Recovered

I have become involved in a breast-feeding support group and I attend classes to promote breast-feeding. I enjoy supporting these mothers in my community.

I don't let trivial things get

> A funny thing happened to me when I had postpartum depression. I put dirty underwear in the toilet instead of the hamper. Then I flushed!
> —Marianne, 36, At-Home Mom
> Ontario, Canda

me down anymore. I try to enjoy each new day for its experiences. My husband and I are much stronger as a couple. Although we still argue, we compromise more readily and talk out our differences.

⤳ TALYA ⤲
36, CURRICULUM DESIGNER
ILLINOIS, USA

I just didn't know it would be so hard to take care of a baby, house, husband, and myself. I felt completely overwhelmed. Every mother I knew seemed able to handle all the demands. They just made me feel more inadequate. My husband and I argued quite a bit. He was hesitant to take an active part in caring for our daughter, but criticized everything I did. He was also critical of my inability to keep the house clean since I wasn't working.

Everyone expected me to "snap out of it." Anyone I mentioned my feelings to thought I was either feeling sorry for myself or thought I was jealous of all the attention the baby was getting. I started to fall apart one month postpartum. I wanted to hide in bed all day. I thought if I could just catch up on my sleep I'd be able to handle everything. The demands of being a new mother seemed so huge, like a mountain or skyscraper. My moods would change at lightning speed and my emotions were out of control.

I cried everywhere, including the grocery store, the car, at the doctor's office. I'd hyperventilate, shake, pace, and scream. I was totally exhausted. My husband would be incredulous when he came home from work and the housework wasn't done. I was lucky to get out of my pajamas most of the time. I used to be an avid reader, crafter, and seamstress. After the baby was born, I lost interest in everything but sleep. Everyone expected me to be my normal, upbeat, overachieving self, and I didn't want to let anyone down, so I avoided everyone.

I never felt I would hurt my baby, but I wanted to hurt my husband for being so unaffected. He just went on with his normal life, without interruption, and it made me furious. My life was in pieces. I couldn't make him understand how I felt. He thought I overreacted to everything, and threatened to leave me and take the baby if I didn't get my act together. So I was in constant fear that my husband wouldn't think I could handle the baby.

I was afraid of my baby not getting enough to eat, getting sick, getting hurt or choking or dying of SIDS. I couldn't relax and enjoy anything. I was constantly agitated. Eventually I wanted to die. I was so disappointed in myself that I just wanted to rid the earth of the mess I had become.

I never sought professional help or medication. I didn't look for a PPD recovery group because I believed my husband would have thought I was seriously imbalanced and would have filed for divorce. He wouldn't tolerate a wife who was "damaged goods." Eventually, I just came to realize that my daughter needed me to take care of her, and if my husband didn't think I was good enough then I could live without him. The more I took charge of my life, though, the better he and I got along.

> Create a "retreat" for yourself. Keep a desk with candles, a journal, music, magazines, books, and paint brushes in a favorite location. Let this location be a place of solace and comfort when things feel out of control.
> —Marianne, 36, At-Home Mom
> Ontario, Canada

⟶ PENELOPE ⟵
36, AT-HOME MOM
VIRGINIA, USA

I pictured new motherhood being a warm, cuddly time of resting and snuggling. To the contrary, my baby nursed poorly, slept rarely and only for short spurts, and cried incessantly. I didn't think I'd be as tired as I was or as afraid to get out with the baby. I was overwhelmed with the preparation involved in even simple excursions to the store. I didn't expect nursing to be so painful and difficult and I felt guilty when it didn't go right.

> Consider buying a white noise generator—one for you and one for the baby. It might help both of you sleep.

The sleep deprivation made me dread each day, knowing I wouldn't get to sleep again. I cried every day for months . . . out of pain, frustration, hormonal emotional roller coasters. You name it, I cried about it. As my marriage deteriorated, I cried even more. I lost all interest in sex, believing the baby drained me of all energy. I had nothing left to give and no desire to receive intimacy. I tried to stay in touch with family and friends and even make new friends with other mothers of newborns, but I was not honest in my portrayal of myself. I didn't share how depressed I really was. I felt like I was a failure as a mother. Other moms seemed able to not only cope with but actually to enjoy their babies.

I wanted my husband to feel as bad as I did. Sometimes I'd elbow him or kick at him in bed when I had to awaken with the baby. I envied his ability to sleep soundly—his enviable role of getting to leave the house and the baby each day when I had to stay.

Eventually my husband and I went to a marriage counselor. We were on the verge of divorce due in large part to my erratic behavior and his lack of understanding. The counselor diagnosed me with PPD, and once my husband became familiar with the illness he became very supportive. Having a name to put on this helped me realize I wasn't going crazy and wasn't a failure as a mother. Help was available for this.

Now That I've Recovered

I'm thankful for having gone through this if for no other reason than to help educate others about it and help new mothers in any way I can. I'm happy to say I had no PPD with my second child. I had a support group in place, a doula, and a counselor if I needed them.

‑‑‑ POLLY ‑‑‑
AT-HOME MOM
MAINE, USA

I now have three boys, ages six, four, and the youngest is almost three. My husband has never been supportive. When I would tell him how exhausted I was with each baby, he thought *I* was being a baby. My husband always made sure he was happy. But he just wanted me to clean, work, clean, work. When I was happy, he was okay with things, but never happy with me.

My husband never helped with the crying babies or sleepless nights. I was always the only one up all night with sick babies. Then he'd become jealous

I knew that by four or five P.M., I'd be very tired, very low. I had a standing phone "date" with my sister every day at that time. Knowing she would call me gave me something to look forward to and I could "tell all." I didn't have to put on an act if I felt lousy. She was very supportive and helped a lot.

—Vivien, 38, Health Care Manager
Massachusetts, USA

because of all the attention I had to give each baby. He wanted me to take care of the baby in the day, and sleep with him at night. We grew to "hate" each other.

I had PPD within one month after each of my babies' births. When I went to my doctor's office, they barely acknowledged PPD existed. They just said the feelings I was having would pass, as if they were normal and I should just leave it alone because it eventually ends. So I was depressed for four years.

I got very little sleep. It was very hard to nap since I was doing everything myself with little or no help. I was so tired; yet I had to care all night for my babies, clean house, etc. It was a twenty-four-hour-a-day job, and I was not appreciated. I was grumpy, miserable, exhausted, filled with fears and anger. My husband would never let me just lie down. He made me feel lazy. I was pale. Bags were always under my eyes. I was not at all "bubbly" as I used to be.

A few times I thought about suicide, but realized I would never leave my kids to my husband. Ugh! I finally went to a therapist and psychiatrist. An antidepressant was prescribed. It helped almost immediately. I was so mad I hadn't gotten this help earlier. Then I started doing things for me, not for my husband. I started exercising, going on camping trips, and having fun with my children. Daily goals turned into weekly goals. I even started voice and acting lessons, something I've always wanted to do.

Now That I've Recovered

I am actually more of a positive thinker now. I am more able to say what I feel and I can handle confrontations better. I am an advocate in my children's lives, and they love me. Give your baby lots of hugs and reach out for help if you need it.

~~@~ SHERONA ~@~~

35, AT-HOME MOM
NEW JERSEY, USA

My husband never gave me one iota of support during my pregnancy. He reminded me that if I weren't pregnant we could afford a new car, etc. Comments like that always set me off on a crying fit, although I never let him see me cry. Then before our son was born, I discovered my husband had amassed a huge credit card debt. By the time I gave birth, our savings account was practically gone.

My husband worked odd hours and I still managed to have dinner ready for him when he came home from work. I was breastfeeding every three hours. When I asked my husband to give me a little break and hold the baby when he cried, my husband would say he was too tired to help and he'd go to bed. I was overwhelmed, doubted my ability to be a good mother, and worried my baby had no chance to bond with his father. I started to wonder if my husband had been right—maybe we shouldn't have had any children.

I was so confused. My self-esteem was slowly draining away. I'd cry all day and stare out the window, waiting for my husband to come home. But he'd only take the baby a couple of minutes before giving him right back to me. I started talking to my mother about my feelings and discovered that she and my sister-in-

> Depression comes in many levels. Talk to anyone who will listen. Read books or articles, watch videos, or listen to audio tapes about how to cope with depression. Get dressed every day—no pajama days! Get fresh air—take daily walks with your baby. And don't be afraid to ask for help.

law went through some of the same ordeals. Suddenly, I didn't feel so alone.

I began making trips to my parents' and brother's houses. As soon as I walked in, they would take the baby and tell me to go relax. I even got breakfast in bed one morning! My family was very supportive. When I would go to my parents' house for an extended visit, my husband would encourage me to stay as long as I wanted. But after a few days, he would call to find out when I was coming home.

My healing occurred when I read about PPD to learn as much as possible about the way I had been feeling. Going back to church regularly felt right, too. I started to analyze why I had these problems, so I could turn them around. I started to believe in myself again. I started to take pride in the bond I had with my son. Day trips to craft stores helped me feel better, even when I could not afford to purchase anything.

CHAPTER 13

Single Mothers

Having postpartum depression without a supportive husband is difficult enough. The mothers in Chapter Thirteen share their experiences with PPD as single
mothers—some who live with their boyfriends, some not. They
made the choice to keep and raise their babies.

Once recovered from PPD, their babies would be the loves and
joys of their lives. Whether these women wanted to be single
mothers or death or divorce created their situations, they all gained
tremendous strength and confidence through healing.

MATILDA
24, STUDENT
MONS EN BAROEUL, FRANCE

The three months after my daughter's birth were the longest
months of my life. I was "baby and bedridden." I cried in the
morning when she woke up when I had never even slept. I cried

because she looked like her father and it hurt to think of him. I cried from exhaustion. And I cried when she smiled at me in week six—even though I thought I was not caring for her well. Thank goodness I breast-fed or I don't think we would be so connected now. My depression actually began when I was pregnant. I was sure it was hormone-related.

> Seek out humor in your life. Cartoons, sitcoms, whatever it takes. Laughter really is the best medicine.

Plus, it was also due to my live-in boyfriend leaving me because I became pregnant. My teacher was a sexist who didn't think giving birth five days earlier was an excuse for not going to an exam. One month postpartum, I returned to the university.

I felt suicidal for two days and that's when I decided to seek help. I found it on the Internet. It was the best experience for me. Having contacts without having to go out because I was too exhausted was marvelous. I found my "tribe" . . . mothers who were experiencing the very same things. Some of them would even post a joke, and I started connecting to the world again. I started to recover when I realized that the baby would not suffer from my taking care of myself a little bit. So I decided to do one of my favorite things: I took a walk in my bare feet to watch the sunrise. I finally experienced a joyful cry. I truly realized what a book I had read said—a mother/baby's well-being is more important than the baby's well-being alone. I faced my fears and left the apartment. Every day I'd walk with my baby to buy fresh bread and vegetables. It forced me to exercise and meet people. And eat those vegetables.

Now That I've Recovered

I have graduated from school. I am a new person. Overcoming postpartum depression has made me learn to enjoy life as a whole much better. Talk about your depression. You'll be amazed how many people have been there. You are not alone.

~⊙~ MADISON ~⊙~
21, AT-HOME MOM
QUEENSLAND, AUSTRALIA

My daughter was sixteen months old when I had my son, so I now had twice as many nappies and bottles. I felt mean and guilty because I was unable to spend much time with my daughter. I was a young mother and felt bad when people would give me funny looks. I imagined I could tell they didn't approve of my single status. I never had a chance to start college; as a single mother I was too busy. I knew motherhood wasn't going to be easy, but it was a lot harder than I thought.

I felt trapped in my own home. My new baby was colicky. My mum took my daughter every now and then to give me a break. Nobody knew I had PPD. I would act as if everything was fine when we had visitors. I felt like I didn't even love my son and wondered if I hated him. That hurt the most.

My emotions were so extreme I thought I was going mad. Sleep deprivation made it really hard for me to think or remember anything. On some days I'd cry all day long, on other days I'd be angry. The only constant was my exhaustion and how my body ached. I stopped painting and began to have anxiety attacks; I was terrified I couldn't take care of my son. I yelled a lot at my baby. I ran away twice and felt suicidal.

When the baby was four months old, I was diagnosed with PPD. I found a great doctor who prescribed an antidepressant, which I took for eight months. My mother helped by telling me what was good in my life. The Internet PPD sites helped tremendously.

Talking with other mums in the same situation helped make me feel that I wasn't alone. The best advice was from my mum. She told me the baby stage was the shortest and I should try to enjoy it.

Now That I've Recovered

Now when I look back, I'm amazed I was that person. I love my baby so much now and cuddle him all the time. He is so much happier now that his mum's better. Don't feel like you're a bad mother, because you can't help this. Depression is not a choice. If you feel anger toward your baby and think that you have made a mistake or that you don't want him anymore, just take a deep breath and look at him. Isn't he beautiful! Look into his eyes and imagine what he could be. Realize he needs your love to thrive and become a healthy baby. He loves you unconditionally. Don't think it's too late to have a great bond with him! It does get easier with time. Look to the future and love who you are and who your baby is.

JODI
23, HEALTH UNIT COORDINATOR
NEW HAMPSHIRE, USA

My partner barely touched the baby—only when I forced him to do it. He never woke up at night and stayed away as much as possible. I resented the lack of help and tried to get him to help more, which just drove us further apart.

I felt PPD started when they placed my son on my belly after he was born. It lasted six months.

I was angry with the baby for waking me up and not letting me sleep. I was nineteen then and felt as if I were the typical teen mom who dropped out of college and lived on welfare while the father was pretty much absent and had a history of being in jail. I had an extreme lack of good self-esteem. And I kept eating as much as when I was pregnant, going from a prepregnancy size six, to a post-pregnancy size twenty-two.

I was so tired. The housework never got finished, laundry piled up, groceries dwindled. None of that bothered me; I just wanted to sleep. I thought I was a terrible mother. What kind of mother resents her child? I always called my mother (we lived in the same house) if I thought I would hurt my baby. She would immediately take him and show me what to do. I was jealous. She would just walk in and pick him up and he would stop crying. I did think of killing myself, but I couldn't leave my baby behind and hurt my parents. I never told anyone of these thoughts.

> This is the day that the Lord has made. We will rejoice and be glad in it.
>
> —*Psalm 118:24*

I went to see my doctor about weight loss and she asked if I felt depressed. She was very reassuring and prescribed an antidepressant. I started to gain more weight, so she switched me to another medication. My mother said in just two days she started to see the old me. I took medication for six months. I will be forever grateful for my mother, who was my entire support in helping me recover.

Now That I've Recovered

I went back to college and graduated with a 3.75 GPA. I am married to a wonderful man now, not the biological father of my son. My husband adopted my son. We plan to have a child together and now I'll know what to watch for, and I'll nip any depression in the bud.

When you are pregnant, talk to your family about the possibility of PPD. Don't be offended if someone tries to help you. Don't feel inadequate. It's the hormones, not you.

MARGOT
24, RETAIL STORE MANAGER
ILLINOIS, USA

I lived with my parents and the baby's father lived with his parents. I knew babies cried, but I didn't know they could cry constantly. My baby was colicky. All I wanted to do was sleep. I would lie in bed as long as possible before getting up for school or work. I always felt worn out. I hated school—I used to love it. Now there was no time for anything but school, work, and my baby.

Whenever I started to go out I would feel guilty about leaving my child, but I dreaded going back home to her. I knew I'd never lose control and hurt her—this wasn't her fault. The baby's father rarely visited. All my friends were childless and didn't understand. The only people I wanted to be near were my parents.

I felt like a failure as a mother. Everyone else seemed to deal with my baby better than I could. She never gave anyone else trouble, only me. I was supposed to be a good mother, a perfect student, and a great employee. But I felt totally out of control. I seriously thought maybe I wasn't supposed to be a good mother and considered putting her up for adoption.

I saw our school counselor for four months, but quit because I wasn't getting much out of the sessions. Our family doctor prescribed an antidepressant for me. I started feeling better in six weeks and took medication for a year. I left school for eight months to relieve that stress. My parents were very supportive and helpful with the baby. And when her father left the picture for good, a huge weight was lifted off my shoulders. I found great support for single moms on the Internet.

Now That I've Recovered

I have bounced back from depression. I sure wish I hadn't "missed" so much of my daughter's early life. Find help on the Internet so you know you are not alone. And take advantage of all those offers of help from family and friends when the baby comes. Tell them specifically what help you need: baby-sitting, a meal, or going to the doctor. Not only will this help you, but it will make the person helping you feel their offer is appreciated.

CECILIA
26, AT-HOME MOM
DUNSBOROUGH, AUSTRALIA

Nothing can prepare one for the full nature of rebirth after childbirth: the loss of identity, the change in one's energy level, and the profound, irrevocable loss of one's former self. You do grow into more of yourself and gain so much love and joy, as never before; however, it doesn't cancel out the loss and grieving involved with the immense changes.

My partner couldn't handle our son's crying and waking during the night. Sleep deprivation brings out parts of yourself that you never knew existed. Leaping from lovers into parents is scary. Suddenly sharing the awesome responsibility of nurturing a child when we had never envisioned being in that position with each other resulted in inevitable conflict, freaking out, and heartache.

I had immense guilt over being so preoccupied and self-centered, lost in my emotions. I so wanted to be present with my son, but felt a lot of the time I just wasn't there mentally. I have always been an eternal optimist and a perfectionist. I had such high expectations of myself as a mother. I have to be perfect and amazing. No room for just an ordinary, adequate mother here. I am addicted to being positive and have always tried to surpass negativity and pain. Not good.

My son was already eighteen months old when I was finally diagnosed with postnatal depression by a child health nurse at my son's checkup. I learned through counseling that PND was a physical condition. Knowing that this was not my fault was a huge turning point for me. I did not take medication. I had to learn to relax into it all and not count the hours not slept or the responsibilities of raising the baby. Breathing exercises and focusing on love made a difference. From there I could find power again. I focused on believing that I deserved to feel joyous and free and that I was getting better every day in every way.

Now That I've Recovered

I missed dealing with the public so I set up a business from my home, using my son's nap times to work. Now that I'm more myself again, I have been so much more present with my precious son. I realized that the depression told me to give more to myself . . . to check in with my soul and love the pain away through self-care.

I now realize I can have it all! It is all possible! I can still have time to just be me, plus I can work from home, and I can have couple time with my partner, where we can be lovers and not just parents. Balance is essential and the key to happy, healthy parenting.

--~©~ GWYN ~©~--

33, REGISTERED NURSE

MASSACHUSETTS, USA

Now That I've Recovered

I am now a single mother raising two beautiful, darling little girls. I know when to ask for help when I need it. I am stronger now because I know what true happiness is. I am so blessed for my life and my girls. I realize I am human and can do a lot, but sometimes I will falter. If you have PPD don't let anyone tell you to tough it out and that it will pass. Being aware of your needs is showing strength— not weakness. You must be big enough to say, "I need help." Get help. Life is too short to be unhappy and you have your child to enjoy.

CHAPTER 14

Postpartum Depression with Second or Subsequent Child

With the second child, mothers already know the huge demands of an infant. Mothers who never had postpartum depression with their first child are surprised to encounter feelings of anxiety and sadness after the birth of their other children. They never had these alarming feelings with their first baby, only joy. These new feelings bring tremendous guilt, not just because the mothers feel they "shouldn't" experience postpartum depression . . . but because they realize how this illness is "short-changing" their new baby. After all, their first never had to go through any of this.

Mothers with postpartum depression after the birth of their second or subsequent child also describe what a huge, unexpected adjustment it is. They never imagined all the changes that would take place, trying to manage time with their newborn, other children, and their husbands.

Like so many before them, these mothers will say surviving postpartum depression has made them stronger, wiser, and more prepared to take on life's challenges.

-~©∽ AUDRA ∽©~-

30, AT-HOME MOM

NEW JERSEY, USA

When I compare my daughter's early days to those of my son, the differences are incredible. This is something I will regret for a very long time. I had severe insomnia. I would fall asleep relatively easily and then be wide-awake from one A.M. to four A.M. and then sleep lightly until six A.M. I was extremely overwhelmed. I couldn't keep up with the demands of my house, my children, my marriage. I couldn't even deal with little things. I completely shut down. Couldn't eat. Couldn't cook. I was angry with my husband, with my children . . . with my life.

I cried for long periods. I dreaded waking and getting out of bed. For the most part, I wanted to hurt myself more than the baby. But one night, when she wouldn't stop crying, I had thoughts of choking her. It was a very frightening feeling. I had never felt like that when my son had cried endlessly with colic.

I imagined horrible things happening to the kids and couldn't get to sleep at night unless I had an escape plan for them in case of a disaster . . . be it meteors or fire. I thought I was losing my mind and even considered driving into a telephone pole. I wondered what it would be like to die and not feel the despair any longer.

I went to a therapist to whom my insurance company referred me. Big mistake. He grilled me on all my family relationships, drug and alcohol use. After making me feel totally insane, he said I didn't have PPD. So needless to say, I switched therapists. My female therapist focused immediately on postpartum issues, but I wished she specialized in PPD. My doctor prescribed an antidepressant, and I relied heavily on an Internet support group. They helped me feel less alone, and they offered wonderful advice. One day I learned that some very good friends of mine were finally about to receive a baby through adoption. I felt such overwhelming happiness for them. It was the first time I had felt happy at all in months. I realized then that I could be happy again.

Now That I've Recovered

I believe obstetricians, insurance companies, and therapists need to learn more about PPD, its many forms, and how devastating it is to mothers. Many doctors don't understand the seriousness of our circumstances, and the depths of our despair. All people who treat women need to be educated. All women should have the chance to enjoy their new babies and not suffer from so many debilitating conditions associated with PPD. Too many women suffer longer than they have to because of misinformation, poor diagnoses, and trial-and-error treatment.

MOLLY
35, AT-HOME MOM
VIRGINIA, USA

I underestimated the adjustment from one to two children. I thought it would be easy since I'd already experienced a newborn. From three months to seven months after my second child was born I had severe sleep problems. I became so sleep-deprived that I became paranoid and thought some people told a social worker to come to take my children away because I wasn't a good mother. I had no appetite at all and became almost anorexic. I was too anxious to eat.

My therapist prescribed an anti-anxiety medication to help me sleep. I had my first good night's sleep in months. The antidepressant she prescribed helped calm me down and the medication took about a month to take effect. My therapist asked me to write journal entries for seven days, focusing solely on my husband and children. I found myself scribbling every night and enjoying every minute of it. It helped me realize how important my role as mother was. I was shaping two precious lives and keeping our family going strong. It was as if a blindfold that was covering my eyes for months had suddenly been removed. The more I wrote, the more I realized how important my family was and how much they needed me.

Slowly I began to feel joy again, in even the most mundane tasks. My self-esteem was inching its way back up again. Praying helped me give my worries and anxieties over to God to let Him take care of things. This wasn't easy to do at first, but when the medication took effect and my anxiety level lowered, it became easier. I became thankful for my blessings and began to stay positive.

Now That I've Recovered

I am completely fulfilled and satisfied in my role as a full-time mother. I'm involved in my children's activities and a support group for stay-at-home moms. I'm preparing to run in a 10K race. My marriage was strengthened by this PPD nightmare that we endured.

~⊛ SHOSHANA ⊛~

29, FREELANCE JOURNALIST

CALIFORNIA, USA

Thoughts for a Better Day

I am grateful to our Heavenly Father, who has taken me down this path of self-awareness and self-discovery. I'm grateful that mental health cures are making great strides. I am grateful to my therapist, who is my teacher, my cheerleader, and a great source of wisdom. I am now passionate about helping mothers in the way that I really missed being helped, because I'm now an advocate—a mentor who's "been there."

~~⊙~ SALLY ~⊙~~
28, At-Home Mom
Wisconsin, USA

My daughter was nineteen months old when my son was born. I felt very guilty not being able to spend as much time with her. I felt guilty letting her watch *Barney* two hours in a row. I was always torn every time the baby didn't need me. Should I finally get the dishes done or read to my daughter? Many times I longed for a single day of just having one child again. I thought, "How did other moms do it? Will my daughter feel unloved? Why did we have another baby when she was so young?"

> Remember:
> Feeling guilty is not the same as being guilty.
> Feeling bad is not the same as being bad.

I felt guilty all the time and then felt guilty about feeling guilty! I thought I must be a terrible mother because I wasn't elated with motherhood. My son was more clingy than my first child. I was having a hard time handling the demands of the household, caring for two, and trying to continue my volunteer work. Sometimes I looked at our chaotic house and thought, "I hate this hellhole."

I escaped to my parents' house a lot, just to avoid seeing our house such a mess. I felt guilty because I didn't feel tender and loving toward my son 24/7. There were times I wished he were never born. I felt anger toward him for taking so much of my time. His demands made me captive to his schedule. My emotions would flip-flop between guilt and anger. I worried he was so clingy because he feared I would try to get rid of him.

Caring for two was so overwhelming I always felt exhausted. I had to get out of bed to care for the kids, but if it had been up to me

I would have slept all day. I couldn't stand to be home alone. Everything I saw reminded me of what a failure I was. I used to ask God why He allowed me to be a mom. I felt He had made a mistake—I was too grouchy and tired to be a good mother. I began to wonder if I killed myself and if my husband remarried, would my kids be better off with a different mother? But I never attempted suicide. I feared going to hell. And I guess deep down I believed God would not have put me on this Earth without a purpose for my life.

At nine months postpartum, I went to see my family practitioner. He prescribed medication. After upping the dosage, I began to feel better. My husband and I literally thank God for the antidepressant nearly every day. I learned that what I was feeling was not normal and that I could be helped!

Now That I've Recovered

We've since had a third child. Being on antidepressants made it far easier to handle. As it turns out, there is a medical basis for my depression and the hormonal effects of pregnancy have aggravated it.

I've begun working about three to four hours a week for a newspaper. I work from home—it's convenient and I really enjoy it. If you have PPD, try to take your day moment by moment. Find a doctor you like and trust. There is hope!

~ RONLI ~

31, AT-HOME MOM

MICHIGAN, USA

Thoughts for a Better Day

Remember, if you are suffering it just takes time to work through your feelings. You might need medication. Find a doctor you can trust—someone who understands or is sympathetic. You are not weak because you need help. If you had a broken bone, you would fix it. A broken spirit needs to be fixed, too.

HEDY
33, SALES ADMINISTRATOR
DUBLIN, IRELAND

I knew nothing about postpartum depression. I never experienced it with my first-born. I never thought about the possibility of even getting it and I didn't recognize the signs. This was my second son, but I wanted a girl. This tore me apart—but I didn't tell anyone because I felt so guilty. My baby is now eleven months old . . . I've made a big step forward by even admitting this.

For days after he was born, I had baby blues. But it slowly grew worse. My husband sleeps soundly and never helped me when the baby woke at least twice a night. Then I couldn't sleep in the day because my two-year-old needed me. I was constantly tired. I would have given up anything to get in bed and stay there, but I had two young children. I had thoughts of leaving the kids, but I fought the urges. I cried so much and so often that I wondered: If anyone asked me why I was crying what would I answer? I just knew I felt rotten and the more I cried, the worse I felt.

> Shower and eat breakfast every day. Get outside. Exercise, keep the curtains open, and bring in the sunshine. Open up and talk to your husband. Do something just for you—a crossword puzzle, listen to music, do yoga, or just meet a friend for coffee.

I felt so out of control of my emotions that I lived in constant fear of hurting my children. I seemed to take care of them in a trance—it was just routine stuff and I didn't have to think about what I was doing. Once or twice I thought about driving into a wall and ending it all, but when I got home and thought about it I'd weep because the kids were in the car and I could have hurt them.

My doctor prescribed an antidepressant. He also suggested I open up to my husband about all this, in spite of my fears of losing my marriage *and* sanity. My doctor enlightened me by saying that my husband was probably suffering, too. He was right—and now my husband is spending less time at work and more time at home helping me with the boys and housework. This, combined with my medication, is helping me recover.

Now That I've Recovered

It is so important to talk to someone who has experienced postpartum depression or depression in general. They are the only ones who can truly understand. Talk, talk, talk and don't shut out your partner.

⇢ KELSEY ⇠
33, AT-HOME MOM
MASSACHUSETTS, USA

I felt panicky when the baby was just two hours old. I felt like I was going to throw the baby out the window. I was afraid to tell the nurses or OB/GYN for fear they'd take my baby away or put me in a psychiatric ward. Here I was with the third child I had wanted so badly, yet I became so anxious at the thought of even leaving our house. Showering, cleaning house, and preparing meals became overwhelming. I began to wonder if I'd make it as a mother. Most nights my husband would come home from work and make dinner. I'd cry because I felt so useless and of no value. I also had thoughts of throwing myself out our bedroom window. I knew rationally I wouldn't—but those thoughts were obsessive.

I just wanted to be in my room, where I felt safe and protected from the world. I remember going to a block party when our daughter was four months old. I went through the motions socially—not really feeling like myself. I actually felt like I was out of my body. Through it all, my husband—who was the only one I told—continuously told me what a wonderful mom I was to all three kids. He helped me so much—even though he didn't understand this illness. I contacted Depression After Delivery, Inc., and found a therapist specializing in PPD through them. My psychiatrist prescribed an antidepressant. I hated the idea of taking it while I was breast-feeding, but I was told the benefits of nursing outweighed the risks of medication on the baby, so I continued to breast-feed. Just one month later I felt like myself again. I was so grateful! I went back to church for a "spiritual connection." I also made a new friend at a La Leche League meeting and finally shared my experience with her.

> Keep a gratitude journal in which you list at least five things to be grateful for before going to bed at night. You will suddenly become aware of all the wonderful people, modern conveniences, and simple pleasures around you. Focus on the positive and the miracles of life will unfold before you!

Now That I've Recovered

I hit bottom in terms of self-confidence. Now I could probably make it through a natural disaster. I have coordinated a fundraising campaign for a homeless shelter. I coordinate our neighborhood Christmas food drive. I have a close relationship with my husband! If you have PPD, hang in there! Get professional help. Don't be afraid to take prescribed medication. Remember that PPD is a hormonal, brain chemistry–based illness and not a character flaw or personal defect!

ᜒᜓ Miriam ᜓᜒ
38, Web-Based Business Owner
Michigan, USA

My mother passed away from cancer when our first child was four months old. I feel I suffered from PPD because my baby was a girl. I didn't get the same feelings with my sons. But having my daughter made me think of all the questions I had for my mother: I would never get answers. I grieved over my mother so much with my daughter's birth. I was so lost without my mother—we always did things together, talked every day, and I missed hearing her voice.

Taking care of a newborn was overwhelming during the day. And somebody was always up at night so we were sleep-deprived. Our house was not a happy house. I felt many times as if I'd lose it—but I had to keep going. I felt like my extended family was not there for me at all. I knew if my mom were alive she would have been at my house every day. Things would have been different.

When my daughter was eight months old I was really at my end. I didn't want to be a mom anymore. I didn't want to live. I started having horrible thoughts about hurting my daughter and sons. I felt I was a bad mom: Good moms don't have bad thoughts about hurting their children. I simply did not have control of my thoughts or feelings. When I had these scary thoughts I knew I needed help fast and I told my husband that if I didn't get some help, I wouldn't be there by Monday.

I saw an article on a National Screening for Depression and went to our local clinic. I was referred to a therapist and psychiatrist who put me on an antidepressant and saw me once a week for six months. After two weeks I felt like my body was being reborn. I realized how "dead" I was inside. I had to finally accept the loss of my mother and affirm how much I had in my life: a very loving and supportive husband, three beautiful children, a new house, and a job I loved.

Now That I've Recovered

Like me, you can survive PPD. It may not be easy, but it will be well worth it. You will feel good about yourself again. The best part is that it can be treated. But you must reach out for help. And if you are not satisfied with your treatment, go somewhere else. I know you are probably feeling scared and alone, but you are not alone. So many women are in this with you, but they are also too scared to share. This is very common today and we need to talk about it in order for doctors to see it.

Seek out help where you feel the most comfortable. Learn about your options and go with your instincts. This experience will teach you lessons you will appreciate later on. Bless you always!

---🕮 SIMCHA 🕮---

32, CLAIMS ASSISTANT

WASHINGTON, USA

I remember the nurses vaguely talked about PPD when I was discharged from the hospital. It seemed as if it was a joke to them—they made it appear highly unlikely. But the depression started just three days later. The worst part was the insomnia. I am still emotionally scarred from this.

I was so exhausted I didn't think I could ever care for three children. I was suicidal, but never hospitalized. Fortunately, I went to talk to my pastor. His wife, who is a therapist, counseled me that night. I actually slept and felt a little hope the next morning. I relied upon my pastor's wife and another therapist. They both saw me through the worst and kept me from going off the deep end.

My doctor prescribed medication that helped me recover. What also got me through day-to-day was the knowledge that God loved me. I read my Bible and listened to Gospel music. I prayed and poured my heart out to God. I yelled at Him for letting me have PPD. I cried and begged him to rescue me. I wrote in my journal until my head was empty and then I would write some more. And when I couldn't fall asleep in my bed, I would get on the floor and go to sleep—I think because there was less pressure there to fall asleep. In my head I thought the bed was for sleeping and the floor was for walking. If I lay on the floor I didn't *have* to sleep. It worked every time!

Now That I've Recovered

I still have my job—hooray! In fact, I got a raise and a promotion. I'm grateful for my life and the ability to think straight again. I have made friends with people I would not normally have made friends with before. I deeply relate to depressed people now and would do anything to help them. I'm more compassionate and understanding and I help lead a PPD website community.

I'm grateful to God that I made it through this. Don't be afraid of antidepressants. They are like the links that fix a broken bridge. You can get from one side to another (and recover) once the gap is filled. It may take several medications before you find the right one for you. You are not helpless when you ask for help. You are wise! You can heal. There is hope.

⌐◎ LEZAH ◎⌐
31, STUDENT
MISSOURI, USA

We were living in Israel in a very tiny seven-hundred-square-foot house. I had four children under the age of five. My husband's job kept him away for long hours at a time. Our home was in a remote area with no one nearby to help me. My PPD began one month after childbirth and lasted for five months.

I had insomnia. Food had no taste to me and I lost my appetite. I definitely became irrational from sleep deprivation. I suffered anxiety attacks and began having occasional thoughts about suicide.

I joined a PPD support group, and although I wasn't able to actually attend meetings, the group leader and many members spoke to me often on the telephone. I also sought counseling with a number of prominent rabbis. I shared with them that in addition to living with the stress of a number of small children in a remote Israeli settlement, with no extended family, I knew I wanted to go back to school to become a midwife.

As an orthodox Jew, having a large number of children is the norm, so I felt a lot of social pressure to defer my desires until my children were older. But hitting bottom with PPD made me face these issues. The rabbis told me to go back to school immediately, so we made plans to move back to America.

When my period returned, the severe depression seemed to magically lift. I think this all had a strong hormonal component, but I can't explain why I only had PPD after one birth and not the others.

Now That I've Recovered

I see now that it is much more beneficial for my children to have a happy, fulfilled mommy than one who is denying her nature and sacrificing her desires on the altar of parenthood.

⁓⊙ HILDA ⊙⁓

37, REGISTERED NURSE

PENNSYLVANIA, USA

I never felt overwhelmed or stressed when I brought home a new baby. But I did feel a little guilty that there was another child that had to share my time. I felt very much at ease as a new mother. I didn't have much trouble sleeping, but I usually couldn't nap because of the other children.

With the sixth child, however, I was very emotional. I cried all the time about anything or nothing at all. I felt more exhausted with my sixth. It was very hard to get out of bed. I withdrew from my family and friends, although I knew I really needed them. I didn't feel like doing anything—even playing with my children.

When my baby was four weeks old, a terrible thing happened. It's still so hard for me to think about it. My son and I were in the mall for thirty minutes when I suddenly remembered the baby was in the car. I ran to the car and found him asleep, but it was very hot that day so I put him to my breast and turned on the air conditioner. I don't think I'll ever be the same because of what I did. I also thank God every day that my baby was all right.

From that point on, I was always so worried. When traveling with the children I'd check and double check all the seats in the car. I limited the places I'd go with them by myself. I never had any negative feelings toward them; however, I knew that it happened with some mothers with PPD and I tried to stay conscious of how I was feeling.

My midwife set up an appointment for me with a psychiatrist who prescribed medication. I relied on my midwife, husband, and family, as well as many friends, who were so supportive. Going back to work also helped me to keep my mind off things. What things, I'm still not sure. There was never any logical reason for any of it.

Now That I've Recovered

It feels good to feel like myself again and to enjoy being with my family. Don't hide your feelings. Go for help and know that there will be an end to these feelings. Often, mothers feel so guilty for feeling so unhappy at such a wonderful time in their lives but they need to realize that hormones are a big factor.

Thoughts for a Better Day

I wish I could say that I found something to make the depression and anxiety go away. But I haven't. The only thing that pulled me through was time. Time to get to know my son. Time to adjust my preconceived notions of motherhood. Time to learn to take things one step at a time, and definitely not one day at a time—that was too much to handle. Time to learn that formula is not going to make him stupid, and it is not going to make me a failure. Time to learn that trusting in God is the only answer, and that He will pull me through.

My son is nine months old now and the pride and joy of my life. He is my single greatest accomplishment in the world. I can't imagine life without him. He wakes me every morning with a beaming smile. There isn't a single day that I don't remember the pain of postpartum depression. But thank God I am past it now. How precious he is to me!

—Joni, 29, At-Home Mom
Indiana, USA

CHAPTER 15

Postpartum Depression with Each and Every Child

Following are stories from mothers who endured postpartum depression with every child—sometimes three, four, five times or more. This is especially inspiring to me, and I'm sure to all of us who've been through it—just once!

Postpartum depression has been described as a truly "hellish" experience . . . a terrifying journey through maternal mental illness. We've been warned that mothers who've had it once are more likely to get it again with another pregnancy, so it is understandable that many mothers will refrain from bearing any more children, fearing they could face this crisis again.

The stories in Chapter Fifteen show that no matter how difficult this illness is, it is ultimately worth the pain for mothers wanting more children. These mothers are now enjoying the large families they yearned for.

ᵔᙉᵔ JASMINE ᙉᵔ
39, AT-HOME MOM
NEW YORK, USA

My typical pattern was to have a euphoric pregnancy and easy, un-complicated childbirth, and then descend rapidly into postpartum depression. I would think, "Oh my God, what have I done? How could I ever think this was a good idea? I've made a terrible mistake and there is no way out."

I could not breast-feed my kids because of an unusual inherited problem . . . the milk literally had no way of getting out. The fact that many lactation consultants thought I simply didn't try hard enough did nothing to boost my depressed spirit. When I tried to make friends at the hospital's new-mother support group, everyone breast-fed and I felt like an odd duck. I was on the outside looking in. Reactions of my postpartum depression ranged from my college roommate saying, "Didn't you want this baby?" to my mother-in-law saying, "Just trust your maternal instincts." What maternal instincts? The only instinct I had was the desire to flee.

I had extreme sleep problems and I was fatigued and lethargic—like a zombie. The sadness was overpowering. The uncontrollable fits of crying were frightening. I felt disconnected from reality and unable to concentrate. Conversations were difficult. Life seemed completely dark and hopeless. I fantasized about getting on an airplane and starting my life over, anonymously, in a strange city. I didn't have the nerve to attempt suicide, but I wanted to. I wished often that I would not wake up. With my first three bouts of post-partum depression, I believed that I somehow "caused" or "asked for" or "deserved" this depression. It never even occurred to me to mention my emotional state to my doctor. But the fourth bout was different. I had panic attacks daily. After vowing to never "resort" to taking antidepressants, I did take medication prescribed by my doctor. At three weeks I started feeling better, and at six weeks my positive outlook on life, my moods, my personality—well, I felt better than ever.

Now That I've Recovered

Depression is an illness. When you have it, you need and deserve help. Getting help for postpartum depression provided the start of a whole new life for me. My kids are now twelve, six, three, and one and a half, well-adjusted and unscathed by my emotional state during their infancies. Thank God my incredible husband had such love with our babies. I have four wonderful, beautiful, sweet, loving, amusing, amazing children of whom I'm so proud and love very much. If I accomplish nothing else in my days here on Earth, this is more than enough.

Mia

32, Part-Time Library Assistant
England, U.K.

After our first baby was born I also had a bout of PPD, but I didn't acknowledge it to myself or anyone else. I lifted myself out of it without any help. I couldn't sleep well at night—couldn't switch off at all. I felt trapped by the endless rounds of breast-feeding and nappies. I thought having my first baby was the biggest mistake of my life. The only relatives I told were my parents and then I regretted it because they felt uncomfortable and embarrassed, which made me feel worse. They couldn't relate to being miserable after such an event.

With the birth of this, my second baby, the depression came on very suddenly, about two weeks postpartum. My stomach was in a constant knot and I couldn't eat. Weight just dropped off me and this was frightening. This time I wasn't so exhausted. It was more

> Doubt is a pain too lonely to
> know that faith is his twin brother.
>
> —*Kahlil Gibran*

that I just wanted to stay in bed and not face any of my responsibilities. I just wanted to curl up and die. Yet I knew I'd never actually commit suicide.

I felt this very deep and very unexplainable sadness—very black—as though I was stuck in a pit of despondency with no way out. I felt very, very alone. I felt I had to go through the motions of normal life for the sake of my four-year-old. With this second bout of PPD, I did seek treatment and antidepressants were prescribed. I got in touch with the Association for Post Natal Illness. Through them I found reading material about other mothers' experiences. Finding other mothers who had recovered was very therapeutic. I could have attended a "Monday Mums" meeting, but I feared that meeting with other mums with depression might make me feel worse. I relied on my husband, supportive friends, and the tablets to get me through the second episode.

Now That I've Recovered

I'm a lot more understanding of mental illness now. I think only people who have "been there" can truly relate to it. Surviving this has made my marriage stronger. One tip given to me by another mother who recovered was this: "Don't fight it. Accept that this is you now. Accept that you are ill, just the same as anyone with any physical illness. If you're having a bad day, just go with it. You won't always feel like this. You will get better."

—✺ LAYLA ✺—
35, AT-HOME MOM
MAINE, USA

I pictured well-behaved children with whom I could spend some of my time doing arts and crafts and educational projects. I pictured them playing happily while I did my other "mom" chores such as cooking, cleaning, and laundry. But as it turned out, my oldest child was very spirited and didn't fit into this mold. No one's kids do!

I thought by the third child I was "ready" for PPD—that I knew what to expect and that this time, by taking antidepressants immediately after birth, everything would be fine. But the depression was very severe. I had also set up support—my husband and mother helped me out the first two weeks. Two days after my mom left, I was often crying uncontrollably. I felt completely overwhelmed and unable to take care of any of my kids. I could not make the simplest decisions such as what to eat or what clothes to put on everyone. I wanted to run away and never come back.

Sometimes I just got in the car and drove and thought about never coming home. A feeling of sadness would come over me and I wanted to stay in bed all day and cry. I remember feeling a numbness—almost like feeling nothing at all. Even when I went to the beach, which I've always enjoyed, I felt nothing. I often thought about being dead, but not really about how I would get there. I knew I needed more medication.

The doctor I saw with my second bout of PPD (I did not seek treatment for my first bout) upped my medication. But I switched therapists and this time went to a PPD specialist recommended by my OB/GYN. Unlike the previous doctor, her sessions helped me tremendously. My therapist also reassured me that by having my mom, sister, and husband help with the kids, I was giving them a nurturing environment. She convinced me that by getting help for myself, I was helping them.

Now That I've Recovered

Looking back, I think that being discharged from the hospital forty-eight hours after delivery added to my PPD. If I was okay to go home, why was I already crying so much? I think there's an unrealistic expectation that moms should be "back to normal" by six weeks postpartum. I continue to take medication and I will continue therapy. But through this experience I know what tools and resources to call upon if I ever feel depressed again.

Thoughts for a Better Day

Now that I'm recovered I feel more capable of facing the world with an understanding I didn't possess before. I didn't understand depression of any kind. There was a stigma attached to depression. Now I can see people in a whole new light. I am more positive about my life and the lives that mingle with mine. After concurring feelings of such depression I feel I can do anything, and nothing in life can ever be that bad.

—Brooke, 37, At-Home Mom
Massachusetts, USA

ALEXA

29, AT-HOME MOM
NEW JERSEY, USA

Now That I've Recovered

I'm now the mother of three and I've survived PPD with each birth. I absolutely feel that weathering PPD changes you. It gives you a new perspective on life. My volunteer life is now focused on helping women with complicated pregnancies and/or PPD. I believe anything that helps women recognize, accept, and heal from these very real wounds is a pursuit of dedication and love. Remember, your feelings—whatever they are—are valid. You are not alone.

-⌐☺⌐ Scarlett ⌐☺⌐
24, At-Home Mom
New Hampshire, USA

Now That I've Recovered

I healed from PPD when I accepted that my life would never be the same again. That was good because I had the most precious gift that God could ever give me.

I had PPD again after the birth of our daughter, but I am stronger now. My husband and I came to an understanding that the housework wasn't as important as giving the kids what they need when they need it.

I never went back to work. I feel strongly about taking care of my kids—I created them and they are my responsibility. I am the foundation for my children. If you have PPD, remember to say, "I am a strong mother. I am a strong mother. I am a strong mother." Love yourself and your children because they sure love you more than you know. And when the day comes that they tell you they love you back, your heart will melt and tears will flow. There is nothing more precious than children.

CHAPTER 16

Mothers Whose Recovery Included Hospitalization

Mothers like me—who experienced severe postpartum depression—wondered in their stories whether or not they would be "better off" in a hospital. Prolonged weeks or months of insomnia and those obsessive, alarming thoughts really make you feel like you're losing your mind. On the one hand, it is frightening to face the fact that you might actually be checked into a hospital for mental illness. You worry about the long-term fallout and stigma that could bring. Would a future prospective employer shy away if they found out? On the other hand, when you are at your lowest most debilitating mentally ill state you've ever experienced, you desperately need help . . . and so you wonder if being hospitalized is the right avenue for you.

For the women in Chapter Sixteen, hospitalization was an important step in their recovery process. Had I not been fortunate enough to have both my parents' support around the clock for several weeks, watching over me (while my medication was beginning to take effect) I would have wanted the same course of action.

Like all the mothers in this book, the endings to these mothers' stories are joyful . . . all fully recovered, all loving their babies and their lives. Many of the stories I received of women who were hospitalized came from mothers who resided in the U.K. or Australia. As postpartum depression gains attention in the U.S.A., perhaps we will learn more about the special mother/baby units in the hospitals of these countries, and make them more available here.

RUTH

46, AT-HOME MOM

HAWAII, USA

The sleep deprivation from PPD caused me to have weird, paranoid thoughts. I felt so worthless—like I didn't deserve to live in my home with my family and I should live on the streets and earn my keep "on my back" instead. It was horrible. And I really understood how easily a person could end up on the streets and remain stuck there. That's not what happened, but it seemed so very easy that it could be me. I understood how someone so desperate to survive might put their children in horrid situations, also for self-survival.

> For God hath not given us the spirit of fear, but of power, and of love, and of a sound mind.
>
> —2 Timothy 1:7

I was hospitalized and appointed a psychiatrist. This was in the early '90s. . . . I was treated in a general depression group. It wouldn't be until four years later—after I recovered—that I found out about PPD. That was from my own research on the Internet. The PPD description fit like a latex glove. The medications I started while in the hospital helped and eventually I was discharged. I hired a regular baby-sitter, who was very helpful, and I relied on my husband and family to help watch my kids while I might have time and space to nap and catch up on sleep.

Now That I've Recovered

I've become a parent-group facilitator trainer for a parent support group, and I'm active in our PTA. I recently spoke about my PPD experience at a conference. It was the first time I'd really spoken about it with anyone in depth. With Oprah talking about PPD I felt much more comfortable speaking out. I felt if it was on her show, we could talk about it.

Trust in your own instincts. If you are reading about PPD and it feels like it fits you, you are probably right no matter what others tell you. Take a list of your PPD symptoms to the doctor. They are not well-educated about PPD yet. I rarely ever took an aspirin before PPD. I was scared of taking antidepressants or anything else for that matter. Now I really must say: Try the medication! And search for PPD chats or boards on the Internet. There are some very understanding women there.

~ ROCHELLE ~

46, PART-TIME CASHIER

VIRGINIA, USA

You know that feeling you get when a car pulls out in front of you and barely misses hitting you? Butterflies swarm in the pit of your stomache. Multiply that anxiety by a thousand and that's how I felt just ten days postpartum. I was so agitated I couldn't sit still—even after my husband made me stop cleaning and folding laundry and just soak in a hot bath with a little wine while he prepared dinner. I still couldn't relax. I couldn't sleep.

My mother, who had stayed with me the first week, came back to help because she knew something was very wrong. I was confused, at times overconcerned and then underconcerned, about my son. At my two weeks postpartum checkup, my doctor advised me to see a psychiatrist. He prescribed medications.

I started having violent episodes, kicking and punching, then inevitably sobbing. I confessed my suicidal thoughts to my husband. At a visit to my parents' home, I became violent again and my husband and father took me to the emergency room. From there I was admitted to the hospital's mental health unit. I had to give an entire past history to the doctors, in front of my father, including my past illegal drug use. As hard as that was to do, it proved to me how bad things had gotten and how much I wanted help.

My baby went to live with my sister-in-law and I truly thought I'd never see him again. In the hospital, no one else had PPD. Everyone kept telling me that depression was depression, but I couldn't relate. I only wanted to help everyone else with their illnesses. I felt like the other patients and therapists just couldn't understand this PPD. It wasn't the same as theirs. My psychiatrist switched my medications. These new pills made me begin to feel better six weeks later, but while I was hospitalized I didn't sleep well. Many people were worse than I was, some locked up, some undergoing shock therapy. I'm glad I was only there one week.

After I was discharged, my husband alternated with my mother or father to be with me. I attended PPD support groups and I called mothers on a telephone support list from Depression After Delivery, Inc. These mothers helped me immensely to get through very difficult times.

At nine months postpartum, I finally felt I bonded with my son and truly loved him without excessive worries. How sad to have lost all that precious time with him when he was discovering the world and how wonderful it is. Little did he know his mom was feeling awful and didn't want to exist anymore. Thanks to my husband and family, in spite of my illness, never once was my son unloved. I will be forever grateful for all their support.

Now That I've Recovered

I've since had a second child with no depression, thank God. Don't think PPD can't happen to you. If you are suffering, don't keep it inside. Let someone know you are hurting. If your medication isn't working, tell your doctor. This is treatable. You aren't going crazy. You will get better and feel love for your child, I promise. The only unfortunate problem with getting better is the nasty statement, "It's going to take some time!" How long depends on you . . . and how soon you get help.

⤳ SEEMA ⤳
40, NURSE/MIDWIFE
NEW SOUTH WALES, AUSTRALIA

My expectations of motherhood were quite realistic, as I had worked as a manager of a busy maternity unit, was involved in lactation research, and was a nurse for twenty years. I loved being a mum. However, I missed working. I had become used to a very busy lifestyle and I seemed to need it.

As a nurse, I had read about PPD but did not expect for one minute that this would happen to me. I actually found it very hard and humiliating to seek help, particularly after working in a very caring and giving profession. Here I was a mum, and it felt great that it was actually my turn. But I became insecure, afraid, extremely tired, and unable to sleep. I became unable to carry out even the most basic of tasks. I became confused and disoriented to time and place. I had a dreadful memory, which was uncharacteristic of me. And I cried often . . . uncontrollably.

I lost my outgoing personality and just felt that life wasn't worth living. The only thing that kept me going was my pre-

"I will get better and I will be a better person for it." Write that down on a card and place it where you can see it every day.

cious husband and daughter. My self-esteem and confidence were shattered. I didn't know who I was anymore. I felt paralyzed and became distressed if I had to leave the house for any reason. My early childhood health nurse diagnosed me with severe PPD, using the Edinburgh Postnatal Depression Scale. I was admitted straight away to a hospital with a special PND unit. I would be admitted three separate times for between four and ten weeks each. I had to give up breast-feeding to start the antidepressant that my physician prescribed. As a lactation consultant, I now felt like a huge failure. I had worked very hard to maintain my milk supply since her birth. Words cannot accurately explain my feelings at that time.

Each hospitalization was very helpful. All rooms had suites for the baby, and for husbands as well. The days were very structured, with input from psychologists, nursing staff, psychiatrists, and pastoral care. All aspects of parenthood were covered, along with learning to deal with depression. My therapy included ECT (electroconvulsive therapy) treatments. The support of sharing with other mothers in the unit was freeing. It's nice to not have to walk through this dreadful journey alone.

Now that I've Recovered

My motivation has returned and I'm feeling excitement in life again. I've resumed gardening, netball, and cycling, which I love. This experience has deepened the meaning of my life. I have always had a strong faith, but now there is a whole new depth of revelation. I have a new level of understanding and empathy. This is a great asset for my professional work. I also don't take life quite so seriously. I have learned to loosen up a bit. If you have PPD, please find a good psychiatrist and a support group. Leave routines outside the door and just concentrate on what is absolutely essential. And please explain the illness to family and friends.

CASSANDRA
30, NURSE
WELLINGTON, NEW ZEALAND

I was completely exhausted—even walking to the mailbox was a mission. At my lowest point, I was unable to get out of bed. When I finally slept, I'd have nightmares. I ended up being hospitalized for ten days. This provided great relief for me. I thought surely those people, experts in postpartum depression, could help me. I remember a hospital social worker asked me to state three good things about myself. I couldn't think of one—the depression completely eroded my self-esteem. I had so much guilt and much of my therapy was expressing this and working on positive affirmations. After being discharged, I continued seeing the social worker and psychologist at lengthening intervals as I improved.

As a nurse, I had no idea how important contact with people on a daily basis had been, and my husband had a job that had him away from home half the year. I was very isolated. I thought I would not need to work after my son was born, but found that, in fact, I was desperate to get back to it. I started working part-time two weeks after being discharged. This added structure back in my life. Having contact with adults and using my skills felt rewarding. It was like work was my medication to keep me sane. It took two years before I would choose to stop working. That signaled to me that I was well again. I didn't need work as a crutch.

Time being the great healer, three years later I wanted another baby. I had twins and I didn't have postpartum depression again.

Now That I've Recovered

I am now a child health nurse . . . I visit new mothers. If someone says, "I am having difficulty sleeping," my antenna goes up. I always share my postpartum depression story. We need to support each other as new mothers and be honest when mothering isn't always a bed of roses.

MARTI

37, FLORIST
BRITISH COLUMBIA, CANADA

Having two children already, I knew how hard but rewarding motherhood was. I knew about the sacrifices and changes a new baby brings, yet it all started right when I got home from the hospital. From there it got worse until my baby was twelve weeks old and I was hospitalized with severe depression. I couldn't sleep when the baby slept, but all I wanted to do was sleep. Through the night I had insomnia, overwhelmed with worry about how to keep up with my baby and my other two children. I'd work myself into a panic.

I stopped eating and lost twenty-five pounds. I would cry so much that when I rarely did fall asleep my husband said he would sometimes hear me sobbing in my sleep. Eventually, I lost interest in all activities in my life, including any interest in my baby. I felt detached from the world. It was as if I was in a dream state and things were going on around me, but I didn't care. Also, I had numbing and tingling in my feet and hands. When I had suicidal thoughts, I was hospitalized for two months. My psychiatrist prescribed several medications. It took two to three months before I started to feel better.

I became an outpatient and visited the hospital three times a week, which significantly aided in my recovery. Six months later, I started to feel hope that I would completely recover. I had so much support from my family, especially my mother and an aunt who practically raised my children while I was hospitalized. Going back to work part-time really helped. Working with flowers and being creative again felt good.

> The hotter the fire, the stronger the steel.

Now That I've Recovered

Although I still have my good days and bad days, I realize now that my bad days are just that—bad days. PPD is real. Whether it is a first child or a tenth, there are so many changes a woman goes through after the birth of a child. Don't be afraid to ask for help. It wasn't silly when you asked your doctor about some "odd" things while you were pregnant. Why should that end after the baby is born? Never let anyone tell you, "It's all in your head," or "You just need a vacation." Find someone who will support you and ask for help.

Thoughts for a Better Day

My family, therapy, and medication were what sustained me through this. I am forever grateful for the support they gave me at the most trying time of my life. Sometimes it takes a life crisis to make you realize how much people really love and care about you.

—Sophie, 28, At-Home Mom
Arizona, USA

CHAPTER 17

Recovery from
Postpartum Psychosis

Postpartum psychosis is rare. Mothers who are stricken with PPP need immediate medical attention. According to Postpartum Support International, only one or two per thousand women experience psychosis after delivery, and the onset of symptoms is usually fast—just two or three days postpartum. Mothers with PPP suffer from visual or auditory hallucinations and have delusional thoughts, usually about their infant's death or the baby being demonic.

When I first began receiving stories from mothers who experienced postpartum psychosis, I was not sure I wanted to include these stories. I don't want to alarm or create more anxiety for readers, but I also wanted to validate those who suffer from this and make sure they know they, too, could fully recover with medical attention.

It is unfortunate that the media reports on stories such as that of Andrea Yates, who drowned her children in the bathtub, don't always clearly specify that the mother suffered from postpartum psychosis, *not just postpartum depression*. Andrea's tragic story helped to bring the various postpartum illnesses out in the open. However, this case, like other similar cases, can stigmatize maternal mental illnesses. The public often associates these rare tragedies with the much more common postpartum depression, and creates an environment in which mothers with PPD are reluctant to seek help for fear of being labeled as unfit mothers.

The vast majority of mothers with postpartum depression do not cause harm to themselves or their babies. As more mothers talk about their experiences in public, our society will take notice of just how common this illness is . . . and hopefully devote more resources to recovery and prevention.

─∞℃ JESSIE ℃∞─

34, AT-HOME MOM

ENGLAND, U.K.

After delivery, over the next few days in recovery, I experienced irrational thoughts and hallucinations. I was moved straight from the maternity ward to the mother and baby unit on a psychiatric ward. At that time, it wasn't explained to me why I was sent there. I was afraid they were going to take my baby away or try to torture me in some way. I believed my room number was significant because in a book I'd read that number was the answer to life, the universe, everything. The picture in the elevator scared me—I thought it contained the flames of hell. And I had other delusions.

I was very frightened, mixed up, and confused. I was put on medication and began group therapy, art and music therapy, an affective disorders group, and other activities in the hospital. Initially, the nurses did all of my daughter's care-taking, and gradually, once the medication was changed and I improved, I began to care for her, too.

Eventually, I could go out, chaperoned, with my daughter in the pram. I looked forward to visits from my mum and husband, who both looked shattered from their daily visits and looking after the baby. The next step was taking days out, then weekends at home. Finally I became a day patient, reporting back once or twice a week. This was a big improvement from the twenty-four-hour watch upon first admission, when you are accompanied even to the toilet and you feel like a prisoner.

I am officially discharged and will be on medication for at least two more years. I don't want my daughter to be an only child, but for now I bite my lip while friends have more children. I don't want my family or myself to go through this illness again. They gave us statistics of the likelihood of recurrence, but this illness is so little understood.

Now That I've Recovered

I take one day at a time and accentuate the positive. I'm very lucky . . . my husband, mother, and friends—who could have all taken things so differently—have stood by me. I feel normal again. I have a part-time job and promote the local charity that helped me and helps other families through difficulties. I appreciate freedom and the possibilities for the future.

MIRANDA
33, AT-HOME MOM
KENTUCKY, USA

I felt right away after childbirth that something was not right. I felt no connection whatsoever to my son and wished he would just go away. I had almost total insomnia for the first two weeks. I didn't sleep normally for two months. I thought the whole parenthood thing was a colossal mistake.

Because I had no feelings of love or connection for my son, I thought I was the only woman in the world who had ever felt this way, and I was convinced I deserved to die. I thought I would end up in jail for doing something horrible. All the tasks of new motherhood seemed impossible, a tower of stuff to do that I could never complete.

I couldn't eat much. I gagged on food and vomited it back up. I was not emotional—I didn't cry at all. But the sleep deprivation made me irrational. My thoughts were not logical at all. I kept having thoughts of hurting the baby and was very afraid I would act on them. I couldn't verbalize this to anyone; it was just too horrible to even mention. I was suicidal the entire four months. Everyone said I had PPD but I felt that I was just playing along with that diagnosis and that I really was just a horrible person who should die. I also thought that I would have to kill my son, too, because if I didn't then everyone would see how messed up he was because I didn't bond with him or love him and I would be blamed. (Keep in mind that even while I had these thoughts, I was caring for him and actually doing the best I could.) So, in my totally irrational state, I thought I would have to kill us both.

The intern at the hospital emergency room thought I should be hospitalized but my HMO insurance and the clinic didn't think I needed it. Social Services was called and they checked on my son. When they saw that my house was clean and my son was fine, no action was taken. I had anxieties about every aspect of my life: marriage, family relations, baby's health, financial, etc. It was an endless cycle of trying to solve a problem and then seeing how that problem affected another area, while thinking this was all just too much. Finally I'd give up one worry, only to pick up another two minutes later and chase that one endlessly.

Once I felt better, each of those situations vanished. I could see that they were not really problems. I saw a social worker, who was not much help to talk to—she had no understanding of PPD—but she was on my insurance plan. A few months later I had four sessions with a Christian therapist. She was no PPD expert, but at least she had compassion. My pastor's wife had been through a severe postpartum psychosis reaction and they checked on me every week.

My pastor and his wife and my husband listened to me and told me they loved me. They kept me together. Then, when I visited my mother in another city, she took me to her doctor. I was diagnosed hyperthyroid and prescribed medication to start my period. Within a couple of weeks of starting my period, I felt better, almost completely normal.

Now That I've Recovered

I had another baby—a daughter. I was thrilled to have a vaginal birth after my C-section. I had pretty bad anxiety for four weeks but this time I had help from grandparents for almost five weeks.

By the grace of God, I didn't have postpartum psychosis this time. God took me through the fire and walked with me every step of the way, though I couldn't see it then. I am a much more patient person now. I am also a much less proud and more compassionate person. I thank God for what He has done in my life.

If you experience a postpartum psychosis, it is imperative to get help from someone who is an expert. Don't trust your life with a provider who does not routinely work with PPD and understand all the new developments and all the types of PPD.

ROBERTA
33, AT-HOME MOM
BRITISH COLUMBIA, CANADA

At four months postpartum, my world fell apart. It started with out-of-control, overwhelmed feelings, which eventually became panic, along with palpitations and paranoia about simple things. Many times I'd flee grocery stores with my kids in tow, because I couldn't handle the pressure of shopping and trying to watch the kids.

Unlike my earlier experiences with my daughters, my son's crying set me off into palpitations, cold sweats, and pure panic. I didn't understand what was happening to me and I felt like I was going crazy. I also started to have periods of forgetfulness and memory loss. I would get in the car to drive somewhere I'd been a thousand times before, and have no clue as to how to get there. I could picture the store, but not my way to drive there. Again I panicked.

I began to withdraw from family and friends as my world became saddled with sadness and despair. I internalized a lot, just felt very alone, isolated in my own world. Sometimes, when my baby cried, I'd be overprotective; sometimes I'd become distant, unfeeling, and uncaring. As my guilt over this mounted, I'd try to share my feelings, but after doing so, was left feeling more alone and misunderstood. I didn't understand how I was feeling, so how could anyone else?

When the baby started sleeping through the night, my mind was a busy whirl of thoughts and emotions, and I couldn't sleep. I felt as if I were spiraling down a dark pit, fighting for air. I started having suicidal thoughts. Then, eventually, the thoughts went into harming my children. My irrational thinking was that my children couldn't live without me and I couldn't leave them, so the only "logical" thought was to take them with me. I knew, on one hand, how wrong it was and how terrible these thoughts were, but on the other hand, I seemed to think that this was the most logical, rational decision I had ever made. I knew it was time to see my doctor.

My general practitioner was a wonderful lady who specializes in maternity and obstetrics. She listened to me as I exposed myself in tears to her—just how far down I was. She prescribed antidepressant and anti-anxiety medications. But I was in denial. I felt weak, like a failure for having to go on medication. As much as I needed help, I was fighting it. I did not respond to this medication, so I was sent to a psychiatrist and was prescribed an antipsychotic medication.

> Sitting down and doing something as simple as a crossword puzzle can help you get through those agitated and hopeless states.

My support team watched me carefully and it made sure that I had adequate support or I would have been hospitalized. Usually a very private person, my life was now on display and my medical chart was forever changed . . . marked in red. I was afraid I would become addicted to the drugs, especially the ones to help me sleep since they helped me so much. But I was told over and over—and had to realize for myself—that this was not a weak/strong thing to be fought on my own. It was an illness that needs treatment with medication and support until the mind recovers. It took about six weeks before the medication started to help, and although I still had a long way to go, I started to see light at the end of the tunnel. As the depression lifted, I began to feel like myself again.

Now That I've Recovered

You are not going crazy and you are not a failure. This is a recognized illness and there is help available. I was very much opposed to taking any medication. I am usually a very controlled, together person who doesn't even take pills for a headache. All of a sudden, I'm a walking pharmacy. But medication was key to my recovery. This experience has strengthened me. I'm now better equipped to handle life, to raise my children and home school them. My husband and I are closer for having gone through this.

Don't resist getting help; take any and all support you can. Remember that kids are resilient and will bounce back with some TLC after Mom gets the help she needs. And my strong faith in God helped me through this. I have been able to enjoy my baby boy and have been blessed with a happy, always smiling baby. What a gift from God—I couldn't have asked for a more perfect baby to have while I was in this state.

—❧ VANESSA ❧—
35, AT-HOME MOM
ONTARIO, CANADA

At four months postpartum, what was supposed to be one of the most special times of my life turned into something far beyond my worst nightmare. I had postpartum psychosis. For me, this was the most cruel, twisted joke Mother Nature could play—and probably one of the world's best-kept secrets.

One day my husband watched me calmly pack valuables and clothing so we could leave our home. I felt threatened, via communication on the Internet, that our house was about to be blown up. I also wanted to call the police and warn our neighbors. My husband's cousin, a therapist, insisted that I go to the hospital that night. My five-month-old wasn't allowed to stay with me.

Two men took me in a wheelchair to a room that had signs: BED A and BED B. Somehow I rearranged the letters in my mind to spell out Be Dead. I doubted the doctors and nurses were real. I even thought other patients were reading lines from scripts, saying things intended to shock me or make my mind snap. I was paranoid that they would poison my food. I tried to only consume foods in packages such as yogurt, milk, or juice. I thought the fifteen-year-old roommate of mine was preparing to stab me with a syringe.

After two nights in the hospital, a nurse who came to take my blood pressure said, "You couldn't be more normal if you tried." I should have been kept in there and put on medication immediately, but somehow I was able to convince everyone that I was perfectly fine and since my house hadn't blown up I could indeed go home.

Over the next six months my mind created many worst-case scenarios and then methodically took me through them, presenting evidence to convince me that each delusion was completely real. It was as if terrorists had hijacked my thoughts, and then months later, one day out of the blue, they decided to set it free again; perhaps because I had held fast and not given in to their demands. But while captive, I had been dodging Nazis, police, and death every day. I was under twenty-four-hour surveillance. I could reason that my thoughts were farfetched, but nothing anyone said could convince me that it wasn't real.

I believed I'd die no matter what and I accepted this, although I still hoped by some miracle I would be allowed to live. I was determined to look after my children, take my son to preschool, attend birthday parties, shovel snow, make dinner, and do laundry, as if nothing were really all that wrong. I did many bizarre things, including talking to imaginary spy people. My world had turned into a super spy thriller nightmare.

Eventually, almost everything in my life meant something other than just what it was. I was determined not to give up breast-feeding or go on medication for fear the pills would kill me. But concerned friends contacted a crisis center that convinced me medication was better than being hospitalized again. My doctor prescribed medication. About one month later, as if a magic spell were broken, I suddenly was shocked to realize that those months of fears were not at all real.

Reality took some getting used to. I began to research postpartum psychosis on the Internet. No one told me that becoming a parent automatically put me in the running to qualify for the 1 in 500 to 1 in 1000 chance of completely losing my mind from hormones, crippling my thoughts as severely as the body is crippled by a spinal cord injury.

Now That I've Recovered

If postpartum psychosis were not such a "hush-hush, don't scare the pregnant woman" issue, and it were out in the open, mothers would have a better chance of receiving treatment right away. I hope that the recent increased awareness of postpartum disorders and the magnitude of damage they are capable of will encourage medical research to make important discoveries, aiming toward a disappearing act for this horrible disorder.

The incident rates of postpartum psychosis have not changed since the 1850s. It seems awareness hasn't changed in 150 years, either. Over the past decade there has been an exponential increase in baby gadgets for baby's comfort, safety, and developmental potential. Have we forgotten that a mother has the most important job in the world? The baby's most precious entity is mom. More knowledge of the postpartum period needs to advance, like everything else in our world around us.

~ᖇᚑ URSULA ᚑᖇ~
34, REGISTERED NURSE
ENGLAND, U.K.

Thoughts for a Better Day

Now that I feel I missed so much of my daughter's early weeks, I tend to spoil her now. I admit sometimes I have pangs of jealousy because my daughter is so close to my mother. But I won't let it become an issue because I would not be here now if it weren't for my mom. My daughter and I are slowly getting to know each other. Her school report card describes her as a polite, helpful little girl and I am extremely proud of her.

I am now much more tolerant of people. Never again will I tell a depressed person to simply "pull themselves together." Now that I'm back to work, which has been the greatest life support for me, I'm able to spot depression in my patients at work. The hardest words to believe when you are at your lowest are, "You will recover." You're in the black hole of misery, but it does get better. You might climb a couple of rungs of the ladder, and then slip back some, but eventually—with help and support and medication, if needed—you will climb out of that pit as a stronger person.

TRUDY
34, MIDWIFE
VICTORIA, AUSTRALIA

Now That I've Recovered

PPD is probably the best thing that has ever happened to me. Now I can see that I am aware of my strengths and limitations. It has made me realize how much I value my family and my friends. Don't be afraid to say "no" when you need to. Look after yourself. You will look back on this experience and be a much better person for it. I laughed when my psychiatrist said this to me, but it turned out to be true!

DEMETRIA
35, AT-HOME MOTHER
HONG KONG, CHINA

Thoughts for a Better Day

I'm much stronger now. I've learned to make the most out of life, to really enjoy my family, and to never take things for granted. I spend more time than I used to with friends. They energize your life. I have a much stronger faith in God. I prayed a lot, and He gave me strength to see it through, and gave me a wonderful husband to help me.

Don't give up. Unbelievable as it may sound when you are feeling your worst, it will pass. It will. Just look forward to that day. Also, find strength in books with other mothers' experiences. Stories like these were like a Bible for me. I read survival stories every day to remind me that if they could come through, then so could I. So can you.

CHAPTER 18

Postpartum Depression Mothers with Grown Children—Looking Back

The mothers in Chapter Eighteen provide great perspective as they offer their stories of postpartum depression from passed decades; from a time when this illness was too often unrecognized or ignored. They were so moved by learning about this book that they shared their stories from generations long past. Their wisdom from having raised their babies into adulthood provides great insight and relief that our children can grow up without any scars.

Several mothers in this chapter, and many more throughout the book, were inspired after recovering from postpartum depression to choose a career which would enable them to "be there" for new mothers who might encounter PPD. Mothers became neonatal nurses, postpartum doulas, and midwives. Some created PPD support groups and websites.

Postpartum depression was an unexpected, terrifying shock to experience. But after recovering, many of us are eager to support mothers who will themselves face this illness and need to know:

- They are not alone.
- They are not to blame.
- They, too, can recover.

These three points have become the mantra of postpartum depression support groups and recovery efforts.

⁓ℭ BAILEY ℭ⁓
43, POSTPARTUM SUPPORT COUNSELOR/DOULA
BRITISH COLUMBIA, CANADA

I had dreadful insomnia. After managing to get just a couple of hours of sleep a night, I'd wake with fearful thoughts about accidents and death. Although I cried a lot, I also got so shut down that at times I couldn't cry. I was exhausted, yet in high gear—like an engine with no "off" switch. Then I'd crash and be immobilized and anxious, guilty that the house was a mess and making a meal impossible.

I felt I wasn't interacting, teaching, or nurturing any of the children well enough. At night I would tell God that tomorrow would be better, that I'd do a better job. Yet each day I felt I had failed. I felt tremendous guilt. I had no appetite and ate almost nothing all day.

I went to a homeopathic doctor who specialized in PPD. She was wonderful. And I attended a PPD support group. I met so many strong women who thought this happened to them because they were weak, but that's not why. These women have been giving, giving, giving all their lives. When they had their babies they were out of anything to give, and their early weeks with their babies were affected by exhaustion, lack of sleep, major transitions, and hormonal changes.

I did not take medications until after my first baby was born. I had a student occasionally watch my children, as well as a friend, who owned a day care. I remember I started to feel better when I could enjoy having the radio on in the car . . . it didn't get on my nerves. And my sense of humor gradually came back. I became more present and experienced more joy in the moment, just being with my kids. I prayed a lot and asked for guidance from a Higher Power.

Now That I've Recovered

I've come from a place of believing that I was crazy and defective to knowing that I'm not. I'm just one of the many women who experienced something difficult during their child-bearing years. My husband and I have been married twenty-four years and we are best friends raising three beautiful boys.

I have overcome my fear of public speaking and have become an activist for PPD support. This issue is so important. Be your own best friend. Treat yourself as you would treat your friend. Don't tell yourself you aren't a good mother. You wouldn't tell your friend all the negative things you tell yourself. You can't be perfect. No one is.

Motherhood, like your growing child, is developmental. You are unique as are all the other mothers experiencing this. You will have your own way of getting through. At the same time, you are part of a huge crowd of courageous women—some who came before you and those who have yet to come to this point in their lives.

It may be impossible to believe right now, but good can come from this very difficult time. You will learn many things about yourself. You will learn transferable tools that you can use to assist yourself and others in the future when life transitions come up. I wish you all the best!

~⊙~ RENEE ~⊙~
47, AT-HOME MOM
ENGLAND, U.K.

Before my baby was born I had read about "baby blues" in baby books, but was told that they rarely turn into depression. Postpartum depression was rarely spoken about back then. I knew I wasn't coping with my baby. I felt as if I didn't love him . . . just fed and changed him because I had to. I was jealous that my husband was so good with him and showed him such affection. I wanted things to be the way they were before the baby was here. My doctor told me to "snap out of it." After all, he said, I wasn't the first lady to have a baby.

I continued to worry about my thoughts of wanting someone to take my baby away. I never told anyone these things before. Other mothers seemed to cope and love their babies, but my mind was always racing. I couldn't eat, couldn't sleep and felt like I let my husband down. Everything seemed so unreal. Everyone was getting on with their daily lives. I felt like screaming, "Will somebody help me!" I began having suicidal thoughts, but I love my husband and could not hurt him. My doctor wanted me hospitalized, but my mother said separating me from my baby would make matters worse. My mother's doctor diagnosed me with postpartum depression. What a relief—someone understood! He even told me not to be ashamed. It took four weeks for the antidepressants he prescribed to help. I became calmer and could sleep more. But there was a long way to go. A psychiatric nurse visited me weekly and was a great help. She kept in touch with me until I had my second child. I will never forget her. I loved my second baby the minute he was born, but I still feel guilty about how I felt with my first baby.

Now That I've Recovered

My boys are twenty-four and nineteen now. They are fine boys and we are very close. I am very proud of them. Babies are very hard work. Don't worry if the housework doesn't get done—it will still be there tomorrow. Focus on taking care of your baby's needs and get your rest. When my first boy turned eighteen I wrote him a story about a mum who suffered postpartum depression. I wrote all about how she felt from not loving her baby—the torment and the guilt—the help she received, and the long battle back to being well. I wrote how I hoped he never felt unloved. He asked why I wrote it and I told him *that* mum was me and he was the baby. We cried together. He said he never knew and never felt unloved. I said I was sorry and he said there was no need to be sorry. I felt I had finally laid down that ghost. When I had my second child, a friend told my husband that I was a different person. My husband replied that I wasn't different but he finally had back the girl he had married.

⮜ LEONA ⮞
51, REGISTERED NURSE
VIRGINIA, USA

I was a second-year nursing student and had no health insurance. Whatever money my husband made he spent on himself. Our utilities were often shut off because he wrote bad checks. I lived two and a half hours away from my family. My husband

> To everything there is a season and a time for every purpose under heaven.
>
> —*Ecclesiastes 3:1*

was drafted the day after my son was born in 1968, and joined the air force. He was gone until our son was two years old.

My depression began six weeks after the birth and lasted about a year. I had constant insomnia and could never nap with the baby. I had no appetite, which was good because I had no money for both of us to eat. Formula came first. And it was a good thing I didn't have a car because I walked around in a fog. Driving wouldn't have been safe. I cried everywhere. I failed at a school test and became hysterical. My friends took me to the school nurse, who sedated me. It was the first time I slept in months. I left my son with my parents and only saw him once a month while I finished nursing school. This separation from my baby added to my depression. My friends were schoolmates and were as supportive as they could be. They were young and couldn't fathom what I'd taken on.

I went to my minister and confided to him my thoughts about hurting my baby, or killing myself. He invited me to live with his family. He loved me unconditionally. My recovery began when I graduated from school and landed my first nursing job. By then, taking care of my son became my bright spot.

Now That I've Recovered

I am now in a very happy second marriage. My son is a successful adult who managed to stay away from drugs or trouble. I raised him alone. I own my own doula business and am a community resource in child matters.

I regret that I didn't get therapy a long time ago to save myself and my son from the years of bad choices I made. Seek wellness and recovery. Tomorrow really is a new day—a clean slate. Be kind to yourself—it's okay to make mistakes as a parent, but admit when you're wrong so your children can learn they can fail and still be loved. It's hard to live with a "perfect" parent. Play, play, play with your child. Housework is not important. On my days off, my son and I went sightseeing, fishing, to the mountains, and to Disneyland so often he actually got tired of it. Surround yourself only with people who are good for you and to you. Don't suffer in silence. Reach out and get help!

᨞᨞ EVELYN ᨞᨞

63, GRADUATE STUDENT

ONTARIO, CANADA

My family and friends all thought I was so bloody capable. They thought I could handle anything. An aunt said, "You are the Rock of Gibraltar in the family." Surprise, surprise; I needed help but no one seemed to give a damn. Just because I delivered easily didn't mean that everything else would go so well. A friend said, since I managed four kids fine, what difference would another one make?

Actually, I did think I could manage everything as I always had done. But things just fell apart. I was exhausted and I cried a lot. I lost weight, felt miserable, and my menstrual cycle all but stopped. My husband was not around much. He worked long hours, avoidance perhaps, or maybe he was just focussed on his career.

Why was I feeling so miserable? I was thirty-two then, with four children already. By the time the fifth arrived, I knew what to do. I wasn't overwhelmed with the baby. I was capable of multitasking long before the word was coined. But the weeping spells were indeed overwhelming and I was absolutely afraid to leave the house. I stayed inside for weeks on end. I had allergy problems and asthma attacks. Antihistamines are also depressants, so it was a double whammy for me. I entertained fantasies of disappearing, moving to some strange city, making everyone suffer for abandoning me from lack of support. I was dreadfully unhappy.

I did seek therapy, but my analyst was a Freudian psychiatrist—next to useless in my opinion. There were no good books back then; in those days PPD was seen as a selfish response. Your baby came first, why should we fret? How dare we think of ourselves? We were expected to suffer in silence. I remember when I went to see our family doctor at the end of that year for a cold. He told me he had thought I was the biggest complainer he had ever met until my psychiatrist and allergist sent him reports on my condition. I thanked him for his trouble, walked out of the office, and never saw that "doctor" again.

What did help me was a study I came across. It linked a property in pregnant women's blood to rapid mood shifts in some women and stated that the situation normally righted itself soon after pregnancy. In some instances it did not, and PPD resulted. So I lived with the hope that the condition would "right itself." I never took medication. My husband and I started working on our problems and we took the occasional weekend away. We spent hours talking things out. I also think my mood just started lifting when my raging hormones calmed down. I continued my studies and the more I learned, the more I interacted outside, the better I felt. Learning became all for me.

Now That I've Recovered

I've learned to do "my thing," ignore my inner critic, and now I'm working on my doctorate in education. I've gone on to survive two life-threatening diseases and have learned to live each day, each moment, not anticipating anything. Each day brings joys and sorrows, and these will be different from the previous ones and the ones to follow. Revel in your strength. You will survive this and be better for it.

Ashley

45, At-Home Mom
Wisconsin, USA

Twenty-five years ago I experienced euphoria after birthing our twins. But by the very next morning, twinges of dread crept in when I saw our babies. It occurred to me that since then I have met only one other woman who was willing to share her similar traumatic episode. And as an air force pilot's wife, I've met lots of women! No wonder PPD sufferers feel so totally alone.

"Going home" day arrived for me and my dad dropped me off at our little apartment with the two newborn babies. My husband was in class at the university because I told him I'd be fine. But the truth was I was very frightened. I had heard numerous times, "If anyone can do this, you can."

Guilt and pride kept my true feelings of incompetence stored away from everyone. As the days and nights wore on, I felt a constant dread. It was if an electrical current was always running through my veins. I was tired, but couldn't sleep. I couldn't eat. The weight of this twenty-four-hour, lifetime responsibility was overwhelming. Friends and family who saw my sadness said, "Everyone gets the baby blues." But this wasn't "blues." It was a blackness that would envelop me and nothing could distract me from the feelings of absolute fear and anxiety. My husband gave as much love and comfort as he could, but it was not enough to heal me.

Although I never had suicidal thoughts, I did begin to wish I'd find the babies dead in their cribs. I called my doctor and told him something was terribly wrong with me. The psychiatrist I was referred to prescribed antidepressants. I also was prescribed a sleeping pill. Finally, I slept soundly for sixteen straight hours while my husband and mother cared for the babies. After a couple of nights of real sleep I started to rejuvenate. I believe much of my depression was plain and simple utter exhaustion. I feel immensely fortunate to have come through those terrifying early weeks.

Now That I've Recovered

I once met a woman who lost a sister-in-law to suicide resulting from PPD. I recall someone saying, "Well, that woman must have had mental problems to begin with." That simply is not true. PPD can and does hit the happiest and most stable of individuals. It does not discriminate. Comments like that underscore why mothers are embarrassed and ashamed to come forward.

I was blessed. My energy, enthusiasm, and maternal instincts did indeed return. And I went on to have another child without experiencing PPD. Let people help you if you suspect you have PPD. Your body has been through a magnificent and formidable ordeal while giving birth. You are fragile. Allow yourself the time you need to get strong again with the assistance of others. This is not a sign of weakness. It is wise.

Thoughts for a Better Day

If you have PPD, don't blame yourself for how you feel. Don't ever underestimate the magnitude of the challenge you're experiencing. Applaud yourself for going through it and be proud of your willingness to face up to the struggle. You'll grow and develop from it. Motherhood is a true crucible. You are surviving the heat that melts you and the hammering that bends you into shapes unimaginable. You will never find final form, but you will discover the enduring strength of steel, the breath-taking strength of your own courage and abilities . . . the inspiring strength of you.

—Shelby, 32, Librarian
Michigan, USA

Final Thoughts . . .

I f postpartum depression has touched your life, chances are that like me and most of the mothers in this book, you want to do what you can to help other mothers recover and enlighten the public at large about this serious illness. A great place to start would be Postpartum Support International. Log on to www. postpartum.net to learn about the wide range of support programs they offer. If you are still recovering from postpartum depression, PSI can direct you to many more resources to aid your recovery, including postpartum depression websites where you can seek help and ask questions of other sufferers in "real time." You'll also find postpartum depression support chat rooms and support groups in your area.

Only by getting involved to help increase understanding of postpartum illness will we eliminate the misunderstanding and stigma surrounding PPD. I invite you to send me any feedback you have about *The Mother-to-Mother Postpartum Depression Support Book*. Please visit me at www.postpartumdepression.net.

I've learned so much along this journey, giving birth to this book. I hope these pages have moved you toward healing. In the future, may we as mothers be more understanding of our individual birth experiences. May our daughters (and sons) know more about postpartum illness than we did. As we shine the light on postpartum depression, we'll illuminate the unfortunate fact that it is a natural part of some womens' birthing experiences, and mothers must not be ridiculed and judged. Instead, mothers must be supported and must learn that by seeking help they can recover and become the happy, fulfilled mothers they yearn to be.

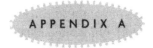

APPENDIX A

The following is reprinted with permission from Postpartum Support International

What Is Postpartum Depression?: Background

Postpartum depression affects millions of women worldwide every year, regardless of age, culture, or socioeconomic status. The symptoms of this devastating disorder range from depression and anxiety to psychosis, which can be mild to acute. If left untreated, the impact upon society includes the breakdown of the family, long-term emotional problems for the woman and her family, and in extreme cases, maternal suicide or infanticide.

Hippocrates described this problem in the fourth century B.C. Modern scientific research began in 1838 in France. In 1980, the scientific community organized the Marce Society and began meeting annually to increase the understanding of the issue and report on their research. Postpartum Support International (PSI) was formed on June 26, 1987, in Santa Barbara, California, USA, to represent the self-help groups that play a significant part in the prevention and treatment of postpartum depression for today's families.

Postpartum Support International: Knowledge

Many women are not prepared for the wide range of feelings they may have after the birth of their baby. They often experience sadness, anger, guilt, anxiety, worry, or a sense of inadequacy. Every mother is different and may have different combinations of feelings.

A MOTHER MAY:
- feel constantly tired
- cry often for no apparent reason
- feel panicky
- worry excessively about her own or the baby's health
- have a lack of feeling for the baby
- have difficulty sleeping or eating
- have problems concentrating
- have frightening thoughts or fantasies
- feel an overwhelming sense of loss

These confusing emotions and experiences can be symptoms of postpartum mood disorders and there is help available.

Postpartum Support International: Understanding

Some comments from women experiencing postpartum problems:

NEW MOTHERS MAY SAY:
- I feel like running away
- I don't feel like myself anymore

- I'm a rotten person, a rotten mother
- I feel like I'm going crazy
- I sometimes think of hurting the baby or myself

PARTNERS MAY SAY:
- I never know what to expect when I get home
- Will my partner ever be the same?
- Something is horribly wrong but I don't know how to help her
- It's tough to live with a depressed person

FAMILIES MAY SAY:
- Will it ever end?
- I'm so worried about my daughter
- Mommy doesn't play with me anymore
- Mommy cries all the time

What Causes It and Who's At Risk?

The real cause of postpartum mood disorders is complicated. Some researchers think it is due to the rapid hormonal changes linked to pregnancy and birth or those with a family and/or personal history of psychiatric problems. Others feel personality and coping skills, if not fully developed, make one vulnerable. Still others argue that lack of social support and information may be responsible. Researchers seem to agree that some of the following social risks may predict problems: recent death of a loved one; economic stress; a recent move; relationship problems; etc. No doubt biological, psychological, and social factors all play a role.

What Helps?

If you are a woman experiencing these feelings, or if you are observing these signs in a friend or family member, contact your health-care provider. A complete medical evaluation, including thyroid screening, is necessary. Psychiatric evaluation may be needed. Psychological counseling can be therapeutic. Sometimes medication is recommended. It is very helpful to become a member of a new mothers support group that will provide emotional support and information.

Most women suffering from postpartum mood disorders realize that something is wrong but often do not seek help. The important thing to remember is that the symptoms are temporary and treatable with skilled professional care and social support. It is important to remember that you will recover.

PSI's Purpose and Mission Statement

The purpose of Postpartum Support International is to increase awareness among public and professional communities about the emotional changes women often experience during pregnancy and after birth.

The mission of Postpartum Support International is to promote awareness, prevention, and treatment of mental health issues related to childbearing in every country worldwide.

Symptoms of Postpartum Illnesses

Reprinted with permission from *Beyond the Blues: A Guide to Understanding and Treating Postpartum Depression* by Shoshana S. Bennett, Ph.D., and Pec Indman, Ed.D., MFT. Moodswings Press, 2003.

Postpartum Depression

15 to 20 percent of postpartum women experience at least some of these symptoms. Onset is usually gradual but can be rapid and begins anytime in the first year after the baby's birth.

- Excessive worry and anxiety
- Irritability or short temper
- Feeling overwhelmed, difficulty making decisions
- Sad, mad, feelings of guilt, phobias
- Changes in appetite, significant weight loss or gain
- Sleep problems—too much or too little; fatigue
- Physical complaints without physical cause
- Discomfort around the baby or a lack of feeling toward the baby

- Loss of focus and/or concentration
- Loss of interest or pleasure, decreased libido
- Hopelessness; thoughts of suicide

Postpartum Obsessive-Compulsive Disorder
3 to 5 percent of women experience at least some of these symptoms.

- Intrusive, repetitive and persistent thoughts or mental pictures
- Thoughts about hurting or killing the baby
- Counting, checking, or other repetitive behaviors
- Tremendous sense of horror and disgust about their own thoughts
- Thoughts may be accompanied by behavior to reduce the anxiety. Ex: hiding knives

Postpartum Panic Disorder
10 percent of postpartum women experience at least some of these symptoms.

- Episodes of extreme anxiety
- Shortness of breath, chest pain, sensations of choking or smothering, dizziness
- Hot or cold flashes, trembling, palpitation, numbness or tingling sensations
- Restlessness, agitation, or irritability
- During an attack, the woman may feel that she is losing control, going crazy, or dying
- An attack may wake her up
- There is often no identifiable trigger for an attack
- Excessive worry or fear, including fear of more attacks

Postpartum Post-Traumatic Stress Disorder
- Recurrent nightmares
- Extreme anxiety

- Reliving past traumatic events. Ex: sexual, physical, emotional, or childbirth

Postpartum Psychosis
Affects 1 to 2 per thousand births.

- Visual or auditory hallucinations
- Delusional thinking. Ex: infant's death, denial of birth, need to kill baby
- Delirium and/or mania

Onset is usually about three days postpartum. This disorder has a 5 percent suicide and a 4 percent infanticide rate.

Postpartum psychosis is a medical emergency and requires immediate medical attention. If you think you or someone you know might have postpartum psychosis, please seek IMMEDIATE medical attention by calling 911, or the emergency police number if you are not in a 911 service area.

Emergency Information

IF YOU ARE HAVING THOUGHTS OF
HARMING YOURSELF OR YOUR BABY, PLEASE SEEK
IMMEDIATE MEDICAL ATTENTION!

Please call 911 or your local emergency number

OR contact the National Suicide Prevention Lifeline at:
1-800-273-TALK (1-800-273-8255) www.suicidepreventionlifeline.org

OR contact The Kristin Brooks Hope Center at:
1-800-SUICIDE (1-800-784-2433) www.hopeline.com

For help through prayer:
Unity Church's "Silent Unity" at 1-800-NOW PRAY (1-800-669-7729)
www.silentunity.org

For contact numbers outside the USA, please visit:
www.suicide-helplines.org
or www.befrienders.org

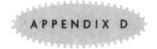

Further Reading

The following books were suggested by mothers who participated in *The Mother-to-Mother Postpartum Depression Support Book: Real Stories from Women Who Lived Through It and Recovered.*

Postpartum Depression: Recovery Books
Beyond the Blues: A Guide to Understanding and Treating Prenatal and Postpartum Depression by Shoshana S. Bennett, Ph.D., and Pec Indman, Ed.D., MFT. Moodswings Press, 2003.

Conquering Postpartum Depression: A Plan for Recovery by Ronald Rosenberg, M.D., Deborah Greening, Ph.D., and James Windell. Perseus Publishers, 2003.

Depression After Childbirth: How to Recognize, Treat, and Prevent Postnatal Depression by Katharina Dalton and Wendy M. Holten. Oxford University Press, 2001.

The Hidden Feelings of Motherhood: Coping with Stress, Depression, and Burnout by Kathleen Kendell-Tackett, Ph.D. New Harbinger Press, 2001.

Overcoming Postpartum Depression and Anxiety by Linda Sabastian. Addicus Books, 1998.

Postpartum Depression: Every Woman's Guide to Diagnosis, Treatment, and Prevention by Sharon L Roan. Adams Media Corp, 1998.

The Postpartum Husband: Practical Solutions for Living with Postpartum Depression by Karen Kleiman. Xlibris Corporation, 2001.

Postpartum Survival Guide by Anne Dunnewold and Diane G. Sanford. New Harbinger Publishers, 1994.

Rebounding from Childbirth: Toward Emotional Recovery by Lynn Madsen. Bergin & Garvey, 1994.

Rock-A-Bye Baby: Feminism, Self Help, and Postpartum Depression by Verta A. Taylor. Routledge, 1986.

Shouldn't I Be Happy? Emotional Problems of Pregnant and Postpartum Women by Shaila Misri. Free Press, 2002.

This Isn't What I Expected: Overcoming Postpartum Depression by Karen Kleiman and Valerie D. Raskin, M.D. Bantam Books, 1994.

What Was I Thinking? Having Another Baby After Postpartum Depression by Karen Kleiman. Xlibris Corporation, 2005.

Postpartum Depression: Biographies

Behind the Smile: My Journey Out of Postpartum Depression by Marie Osmond. Warner Books, 2002.

A Daughter's Touch: One Woman's Journey Through Postpartum Depression by Sylvia Lasalandra. Quattro M Publishing, 2005.

Down Came the Rain: My Journey Through Postpartum Depression by Brooke Shields. Hyperion, 2005.

Inconsolable: How I Threw My Mental Health Out with the Diapers by Marrit Ingman. Seal Press, 2005.

Sleepless Days: One Woman's Journey Through Postpartum Depression by Susan Kushner Resnick. St. Martin's Press, 2001.

Surviving Post-Natal Depression: At Home, No One Hears You Scream by Cara Aiken. Jessica Kingsley Publishers, Ltd., 2000.

Postpartum Care Books

After the Baby's Birth: A Woman's Way to Wellness: A Complete Guide for Postpartum Women by Robin Lim. Ten Speed Press, 2001.

I Wish Someone Had Told Me: A Realistic Guide to Early Motherhood by Nina Barrett. Academy Chicago Publishers, 1997.

Laughter and Tears: The Emotional Life of New Mothers by Libbylee Colemen, Ph.D. Owl Books, 1997.

Mothering the New Mother: Women's Feelings and Needs After Childbirth by Sally Placksin. Newmarket Press, 2000.

Natural Health After Birth: The Complete Guide to Postpartum Wellness by Aviva Jill Romm. Healing Arts Press, 2002.

Depression/Anxiety Recovery Books

The Anxiety and Phobia Workbook by Edmund Bourne. New Harbinger Publications, 2005.

Beating the Blues: A Self Help Approach to Overcoming Depression by Susan Tanner and Jillian Ball. Transworld Publishers, Division of Random House Australia, 2000.

Beyond Crazy: Journeys Through Mental Illness by Julia Nunes and Scott Simmie. McClelland & Stewart Ltd., 2002.

Brain Lock: Free Yourself from Obsessive-Compulsive Behavior by Jeffrey Schwartz. Regan Books, 1997.

Feeling Good: The New Mood Therapy by David Burns, M.D. Avon, 1999.

The Freedom from Depression Workbook: Minirth Meier New Life Series by Les Carter, Ph.D., and Frank Minirth. Nelson Books, 1995.

From Panic to Power: Proven Techniques to Calm Your Anxieties, Conquer Your Fears and Put Control in Your Life by Lucinda Bassett. Harper Resource, 1997.

How to Heal Depression by Harold H. Bloomfield and Peter McWilliams. Prelude Press, 1995.

Mind over Mood: Change How You Feel by Changing the Way You Think by

Dennis Greenberger and Christine Padersky. The Guilford Press, 1995.

On the Edge of Darkness: America's Most Celebrated Actors, Journalists, and Politicians Chronicle Their Most Arduous Journey by Kathy Cronkite. Delta, 1995.

Overcoming Worry and Fear by Paul A. Hauck. Westminster John Knox Press, 1975.

A Season of Suffering: One Family's Journey through Depression by John A. Timmerman. Multnomah Publishers, 1988.

Tormenting Thoughts and Secret Rituals: The Hidden Epidemic of Obsessive-Compulsive Disorder by Ian Osborn. Dell, 1999.

When Someone You Love Is Depressed by Xavier Amador and Laura Rosen. Free Press, 1997.

When Words Are Not Enough by Valerie Raskin. Broadway, 1997.

Women's Moods: What Every Woman Must Know About Hormones, the Brain, and Emotional Health by Deborah Sichel and Jeanne Watson Driscoll. Harper Paperbacks, 2000.

Inspiration, Happiness, and Self-Help Books

The 100 Simple Secrets of Happy People by David Niven, Ph.D. Harper-Collins, 2001.

Chicken Soup for the Mother's Soul by Jack Canfield, Mark Victor Hansen, Jennifer Hawthorne, and Marci Shimoff. HCI, 1997.

The Courage to Give: Inspiring Stories of People Who Triumphed over Tragedy to Make a Difference in the World by Jackie Waldman and Janice Leibs Dworkis. Canari Press, 1999.

Happiness Is a Serious Problem: A Human Nature Repair Manual by Dennis Prager. Regan Books, 1999.

Heartbeats: Encouraging Words for New Moms by Sandra Byrd. Waterbrook Press, 2000.

Help Me, I'm Worried! Overcoming Emotional Battles with the Power of God's Word (Help Me Series) by Joyce Meyer. Harrison House, 1997.

Hot Chocolate for the Mystical Soul: 101 True Stories of Angels, Miracles, and Healings by Arielle Ford. Plume Books, 1998.

How to Stop Worrying and Start Living by Dale Carnegie. Pocket Books, 1990.

I Know Why the Caged Bird Sings by Maya Angelou. Bantam Books, 1983.

Life Strategies: Doing What Works, Doing What Matters by Phillip C. Mc-Graw, Ph.D. Hyperion, 1999.

Meditations for Women Who Do Too Much by Anne Wilson Schaef. Harper San Francisco, 2004.

The Motherhood Club: Help, Hope and Inspiration for New Mothers from New Mothers by Shirley Washington and Anne Dunnewold. HCI, 2002.

Nine Months and Counting: Bible Promises and Bright Ideas for Pregnancy and After by Alica Zillman Chapin. Tyndale House, 1999.

No More Lone Ranger Moms: Women Helping Women in the Practical Everyday-ness of Life by Donna Parton. Bethany House, 1995.

Self and Soul: A Woman's Guide to Enhancing Self Esteem Through Spirituality by Adele Wilcox. Rodale, 1997.

Simple Abundance: A Journal of Gratitude by Sarah Ban Breathnach. Warner Books, 1996.

Talking to God: Personal Prayers for Times of Joy, Sadness, Struggle, and Celebration by Rabbi Naomi Levy. Knopf, 2002.

The Purpose-Driven Life: What on Earth Am I Here For? by Rick Warren. Zondervan, 2002.

The Right Words at the Right Time by Marlo Thomas. Atria, 2002.

A Woman's Worth by Marianne Williamson. Ballantine Books, 1994.

The Women's Book of Resilience: 12 Qualities to Cultivate by Beth Miller, Ph.D. Canari Press, 2005.

The Women's Book of Soul: Meditations for Courage, Confidence, and Spirit by Sue Patton. Canari Press, 1998.

The Worrywart's Companion: Twenty-One Ways to Soothe Yourself and Worry Smart by Beverly Potter. Wildcat Canyon Press, 1997.

To Begin Again: The Journey Toward Comfort, Strength, and Faith in Difficult Times by Rabbi Naomi Levy. Ballantine, 1997.

You Can Heal Your Life by Louise Hay. Hay House, 1999.

You Can't Afford the Luxury of a Negative Thought (The Life 101 Series) by Peter McWilliams. Prelude Press, 1995.

Reflections on New Motherhood Books

The Blue Jay's Dance: A Birth Year by Louise Erdrich. Harper Perennial, 1996.

Child of Mine: Original Essays on Becoming a Mother by Christine Baker Kline. Delta, 1998.

From Here to Maternity: Confessions of a First Time Mother by Carol Weston. Little Brown & Co., 1991.

If Only I Were a Better Mother by Melissa Gayle West. Stillpoint, 1992.

The Mask of Motherhood: How Becoming a Mother Changes Our Lives and Why We Never Talk About It by Susan Maushart. Penguin Nonclassics, 2000.

The Mommy Brain: How Parenthood Makes Us Smarter by Kathleen Ellison. Basic Books, 2005.

The Mother Dance: How Children Change Your Life by Harriett Lerner. Harper Publications, 1999.

Motherhood and How It Has Undermined Women by Susan Douglas and Meredith Michaels. Free Press, 2004.

Motherhood: What It Does to Your Mind by Jane Price. Harper San Francisco, 1989.

The Mother Knot by Jane Lazarre and Maureen T. Reddy. Duke University Press, 1997.

Mothers Who Think: Tales of Real Life Parenthood by Camille Peri and Kate Moses. Washington Square Press, 2000.

Operating Instructions: A Journal of My Son's First Year by Anne Lamott. Anchor, 2005.

Perfect Madness: Motherhood in the Age of Anxiety by Judith Warner. Riverhead, 2005.

The Power of Mother Love: Strengthening the Bond Between You and Your Child by Brenda Hunter. Waterbrook Press, 1999.

The Truth Behind the Mommy Wars: Who Decides What Makes a Good Mother by Miriam Peskowitz. Seal Press, 2005.

Infant/Child Care Books

The 8 Seasons of Parenthood: How the Stages of Parenting Constantly Reshape Our Adult Identities by Barbara C. Unell and Jerry Wyckoff. Crown, 2000.

Are We Having Fun Yet? The 16 Secrets of Happy Parenting by Kay Willis. Warner Books, 1998.

The Baby Book: Everything You Need to Know About Your Baby from Birth to Age Two by William Sears. Little, Brown, 2003.

Bottle-Feeding Without Guilt: A Reassuring Guide for Loving Parents by Peggy Robin. Prima Lifestyles, 2005.

Children Are from Heaven: Positive Parenting Skills for Raising Cooperative, Confident, and Compassionate Children by John Gray. Harper Paperbacks, 2001.

Infants and Mothers by T. Berry Brazelton. Dell, 1983.

Mothering your Nursing Toddler by Norma Jane Bumgarner. La Leche League International, 2000.

Nighttime Parenting: How to Get Your Baby and Child to Sleep (La Leche League International Book) by William Sears, M.D. Plume, 1999.

Nurture by Nature: Understand Your Child's Personality Type and Become a Better Parent by Paul D. Tieger and Barbara Barron-Tieger. Little, Brown, 1997.

Six-Point Plan for Raising Happy, Healthy Children by John Rosemond. Andrew McMeel, 1989.

Solve Your Child's Sleep Problems by Richard Ferber. Fireside, 1986.

Temperament Tools: Working with Your Child's Inborn Traits by Helen Neville and Diane Clark Johnson. Parenting Press, 1997.

The Womanly Art of Breast-feeding by La Leche League International. Plume, 2004.

The Wonder of Boys by Michael Gurian. Jeremy P. Tarcher/Putnam, 1997.

What to Expect the First Year by Heidi Murkoff, Sandee Hathaway, and Arlene Eisenberg. Workman Publishing, 2003.

Your Baby and Child by Penelope Leach. Knopf, 1997.

Comedic-Relief Books

Babies and Other Hazards of Sex: How to Make a Tiny Person in Only Nine Months with Tools You Probably Have Around the Home by Dave Barry. Rodale Press, 2000.

Babyhood by Paul Reiser. Avon Books, 1997.

Baby Laughs: The Naked Truth About the First Year of Mommyhood by Jenny McCarthy. Dutton, 2005.

The Big Rumpus: A Mother's Tale from the Trenches by Ayun Halliday. Seal Press, 2002.

Confessions of a Slacker Mom by Muffy Mead-Ferro. DaCapo Lifelong, 2004.

Daddy Smarts: A Guide to Rookie Fathers by Bradley Richardson. Taylor Trade, 2000.

Driving Under the Influence of Children: A Baby Blues Treasury by Rick Kirkman and Jerry Scott. Andrew McMeel Publishers, 2005.

Expect the Unexpected When You're Expecting: A Hilarious Look at the Trials and Tribulations of Pregnancy (A Parody) by Eunice Glick, Mindee Glick-Garcia, and Bonnie Glick-MacGinnis. Perennial, 1995.

Fatherhood by Bill Cosby. Berkley, 1986.

The Girlfriends' Guide to Suriving the First Year of Motherhood by Vicki Iovine. Perigee, 1997.

The Hip Mama Survival Guide: Advice from the Trenches on Pregnancy, Childbirth, Cool Names, Clueless Doctors, Potty Training, and Toddler Avengers by Ariel Gore. Hyperion, 1998.

How Not to Be a Perfect Mother: The Crafty Mother's Guide to the Quiet Life by Libby Purves. HarperCollins, 1986.

It Could Happen to You: Diary of a Pregnancy and Beyond by Martha Brockenbrough. Andrew McMeel Publishers, 2002.

The Mommy Chronicles: Conversations Sharing the Comedy and Drama of Pregnancy and New Motherhood by Sara Ellington and Stephanie Triplett. Hay House, 2005.

The Mother's Guide to the Meaning of Life: What I've Learned in My Never-Ending Quest to Become a Dali Mama by Amy Krause Rosenthal. Rodale Press, 2001.

The Mother Trip: Hip Mama's Guide to Staying Sane in the Chaos of Motherhood by Ariel Gore. Seal Press, 2000.

The Same Phrase Describes My Marriage and My Breasts: Before the Kids, They Used to be Such a Cute Couple by Amy Rosenthal. Andrew McMeel Publishers, 1998.

About the Author

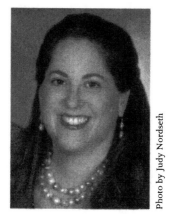

Sandra Poulin grew up in Milwaukee, Wisconsin, the youngest of six children. She received her Bachelor of Arts degree from the University of Wisconsin-Milwaukee, majoring in mass communication.

Now in her twenty-fourth year as a radio broadcast sales executive, her awards include the "Award of Excellence" from the Dallas Chapter of American Women in Radio and Television (AWRT).

She resides in Dallas, Texas, with her husband, Tim, and daughter, Rachel Lilly.